A Quick Understanding on

What Doctors Are Prescribing:

Pharmacology for Everyday People &
Finding Alternative Medications

Arthur Wang

A Quick Understanding on What Doctors Are Prescribing: Pharmacology for Everyday People and Finding Alternative Medications by Arthur Wang

http://what-doctors-are-prescribing.blogspot.com

Copyright © 2010 by Arthur Wang. All rights reserved

Published by Arthur Wang

First Edition on January 2010

Although the author and publisher have exhaustively researched all sources to ensure the accuracy and completeness of the information contained in this book, we assume no responsibility for errors, inaccuracies, omissions or any other inconsistency herein. Readers should consult a practicing medical professional for their medical conditions.

All rights reserved by the author. No part of this publication may be reproduced, stored in a retrieval system, or transmitted in any form or by any means, electronic, mechanical, photocopying, recording or otherwise, without the prior permission of the publisher and/or author.

Library of Congress Control Number: 2010904210
ISBN-13: 978-0-9826347-0-7
ISBN-10: 0-982-63470-6

Printed in the United States of America

I dedicate this book

to my grandparents and parents who inspired me to learn science

to my love, Iris, who supports me tirelessly in every way and shares the dream with me

to my son, David, who gives me endless surprises and inspirations

to my friends and love ones, who have faith in me.

Table of Contents

Introduction

Getting prescription drugs after visiting a doctor has become a ritual for most of people nowadays since people are accustomed to think that taking drugs are an effective way in curing medical problems. For some people, there may be some psychological reasons behind taking medicine. Some patients show urge to obtain prescription even if there is no need. In contrast to these patients, there are patients who strongly oppose taking any medications because of their side effects or they simply want to avoid taking them if they have the options.

In order to maximize the therapeutic effects and minimize the side effects of a drug, we need to learn more about how drugs interact with our body. There are many drugs which act similarly but one drug may be more suitable than the other even though these drugs are treating the same disease.

The study of the effects of drugs on the body or pharmacology may be a complicated subject for many people. This book intends to describe pharmacology to the everyday people in a concise and easily understand manner. The more you understand how drugs interact with your body, the more help you can offer to yourself. Best of all, you can communicate with your doctors easier and receive more supports from your doctors. In addition, you may discover there are other medications available to you or to your love ones beside what doctors prescribed.

Remember the information contain in this book should NOT be used as a substitute for consultation with practicing medical professional.

1

Quick Understanding on Pharmacology

In this section, I will try to bring you up to speed to learn everything about drugs even if you never thought about you can do it or thought the subject of drugs is too complicated to understand. I guarantee you that before finishing one third of the book, you may think that pharmacology is easier than you thought after all. When specific words or names of drug reappear in the subsequent pages, I will always identify with section number previously you have seen. In this way, you can easily reference back to what you have learned and gain new information from it. Therefore, I highly recommend you to read it sequentially for the first time and use it as an invaluable reference in the future.

1.1 How a drug is born?

Substances that used to treat illness are commonly called drugs. As people discovered new uses in old drugs or found new drugs, the list of drugs will be updated from time to time. In the United States, the drugs are approved by FDA, and it takes on average 12 years and over $350 million dollars to get new drug from the laboratory onto the pharmacy shelf. Before a company that developed a drug can submit to FDA for review, it needs three and a half year of laboratory testing. If the FDA accepts to review the new drug, it will enter three phases of clinical trials. The post-approval trials that are sometimes a condition attached by the FDA to the approval and this will be known as the Phase 4 Trial or Post Marketing Surveillance Trial.

The Process of New Drug Development

Drug Discovery
Synthesis, Development & Screening: 2-10 years

Pre-Clinical Testing
Lab and Animal Testing: 3-5 years

(Phase I ~ Phase III: 3 -5 year)
Phase I
Determine safety and dosage

Phase II
Assess efficacy and side effects

Phase III
Monitor efficacy and adverse reactions to long-term use

NDA (New Drug Application) Filling: 1-3 years

FDA Review and Approval

Phase 4
Post-marketing Studies and product surveillance:
4-10 years

1.2 Potency and Efficacy

A drug's effects can be evaluated in terms of strength (potency) or effectiveness (efficacy).

Potency refers to the amount of drug (usually expressed in milligrams) needed to produce an effect, such as relief of pain or reduction of blood pressure. For instance, if 5 milligrams of drug A relieves pain as effectively as 10 milligrams of drug B, drug A is twice as potent as drug B.

Efficacy refers to the potential maximum therapeutic response that a drug can produce or the power to produce a therapeutic effect.

1.3 Four Major Effects of Drug

1. Effect at Cellular Level

There are many receptors on the surface of a cell, and you can think it like a dashboard on your car. Once a substance or a drug binds to a specific receptor, it is similar as pressing a button on the dashboard. This action triggers a specific action to take place inside the cell via a relay activity or cascade pathway.

2. Acting as Enzyme Inhibitors

Since the cellular activities are all biochemical reactions and most of time it involves a middle man in the process, and we can think that enzyme is that middle man who is assisting the reaction from A to B. In this case, the drug is acting by inhibiting the middle man temporarily or permanently. Consequently, the reaction or the pathway is blocked and then it can not be carried out at all. So depending on the concentration of the drug substance, the activities of converting from A to B is dramatically reduced in the cells. For example, if you have 100 enzyme X molecules, and 50 drug molecules, the activities of enzyme X will be reduced in 50% since 50% of enzyme X is being blocked.

3. Effect on DNA (Anti-Metabolites)

This type of drugs are usually targeting for cancerous cells which they inhibit the synthesis of DNA or RNA and as a result, the cancer cells cannot be multiplied or grown. For example, folic acid (or folate) is a cofactor* in DNA replication and biosynthesis of purines** and DNA repair. There are drugs inhibit folic acid or known as the folic acid antagonists***, such as methotrexate and 5-fluorouracil (5-FU), can inhibit the enzymatic pathways for biosynthesis of nucleic acids by substituting for folic acid and this results in shutting down the production pathway and thus kills the cancer cells.

*Cofactor is a helper substance that assists the process.
** Purines are one of components that made up DNA strand
*** When a substance is classified as antagonists to a specific receptor which means that this substance can bind the receptor but the receptor does not send signal. Thus, it inactivates the receptor as a result. If it is antagonist to an enzyme, it will inactivate the enzyme.

4. Physical and Chemical Changes in organs

There are drugs that change the chemistry of particular organ and thus reverse the ill condition in patient's body. For example, antacid can increase the pH level in stomach and thus alleviate the discomfort results in acid over flux.

1.4 Receptors

The concept of receptor is used to explain how a drug works by interacting with cells. However, only a few receptors are actually been identified today. We can use the receptor as a virtual structure in order to understand how drug works in the body and obtains the desire therapeutic effect. We can think that there are two types of receptors. Depending on the roles of receptors, it can act as an activator or an inhibitor. When the receptor is acting as an activator, it increases the production of certain metabolites via a number of biochemical pathways. In contrast, when it acts as an inhibitor, it blocks the production of certain metabolites.

The idea of receptor is not necessary always locating outside of cell, but also in inside of cell. Some drugs like steroid are fat soluble and it can travel thru cell membrane, which is made of fat soluble substance. In addition, most of drugs are water soluble that cannot travel into cell readily, so it is theoretical that there are some receptors or transporters that facilitate the entry of these substances. The concept of receptor helps us to understand how drug may work inside the body.

There are three major types of receptors located outside of cell which are responsible for the entry or the action of the drugs.

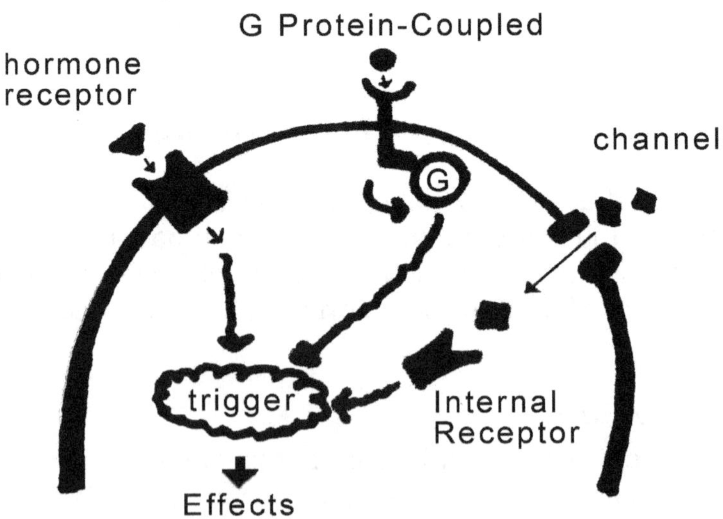

1. Channels

There are a variety of channels presenting in cell membrane: Chloride (Cl^-), Potassium (K^+), Sodium (Na^+), Calcium (Ca^{2+}), and Proton. Drugs may interact with certain receptors and results in opening certain channel directly or indirectly. Once one of these types of channels is being opened, ions rush into cell and trigger some biochemical pathways and results the therapeutic effect that the drug desired.

2. G protein-coupled receptor (GPCR)

Many drugs are using this receptor to relay the therapeutic effect. You can think GPCR as our light switch, turning on and off by changing its knob. In a similar fashion, by binding the receptor, it will change its conformation, and thus triggering some processes just like turning on the light switch, and it will be reversed or turned off if certain conditions met. For example the cause of chronic myelogenous leukemia (CML) is that one of the GPCRs called tyrosine kinase is stuck with "ON" position so the cancer cells grow uncontrollably. (We will discuss this in more detail in section of Medication for Cancer)

3. Hormone receptors

There are hormone receptors where it will trigger the release or block the release of certain hormone. If a molecule triggers it, then we called it, an agonist, and if it blocks or stops the hormone production, we called it, antagonist (as discussed in 1.3.3).

There are other receptors that located inside of cell.

1. Acetylcholine receptors or ACh

There are 2 major types of acetylcholine receptors in the body: nicotine Ach receptors (nAChRs) and muscarine Ach receptors (mAChRs). These receptors were named by the name of the molecule they discovered to bind to that receptor. For example, nACh receptor is also called nicotine receptor since it was discovered that nicotine can bind to that receptor. In this case, nicotine was mimicking naturally occurring substance, acetylcholine, to bind to that receptor.

2. Hormone receptors located in organs

The adrenal glands located near kidney can secret catecholamines* from its adrenal medulla. This secretion can enter bloodstream and reach the target organ where they have adrenergic receptors on their surface. Depending on types of receptors: Alpha1, Alpha 2, Beta 1, Beta 2, it will have different effects on the organ itself. For example, via beta receptors, it increases the rate and force of contraction of the heart muscle.

* Catecholamines are referred as a big group of substances secreted by the adrenal glands. Examples of Catecholamines are dopamine, epinephrine, and norepinephrine.

3. Serotonin (5-Hydroxytryptamine, 5HT)

Serotonin is a type of amino acid found in the GI* tract (90%), platelets (9%), and nervous system (>1%). It acts as a neurotransmitter where it will affect sleep, mood, intestinal movements, and cognitive function. When it is in the blood, it also helps to regulate blood clotting.

*Gastrointestinal Tract is abbreviated as GI tract.

1.5 Synapses

A synapse is a space or junction between 2 terminals of a neuron and the receiving cell. The carrier moves from one neuron to another neuron is called the neurotransmitter. This is where the action or the signal transmission is taking place. If you are familiar with how internet works, the synapse is similar to a hop. The target cell can be a muscle fiber or another neuron. Drugs will be working directly on synapse area, or indirectly by increasing or decreasing of production of a particular neurotransmitter.

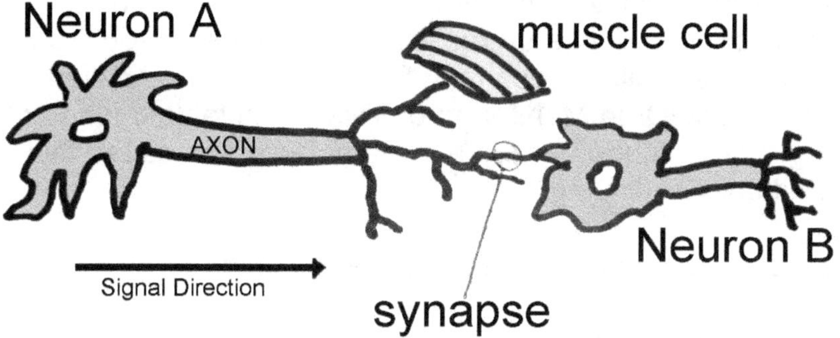

When a nerve impulse is initiated by the release of voltage-gated ion channels embedded in the membrane of a neuron, the action potential is traveled like waves of voltage along the axons of neurons. Thus, this is how signal is transmitted from one neuron to the next neuron.

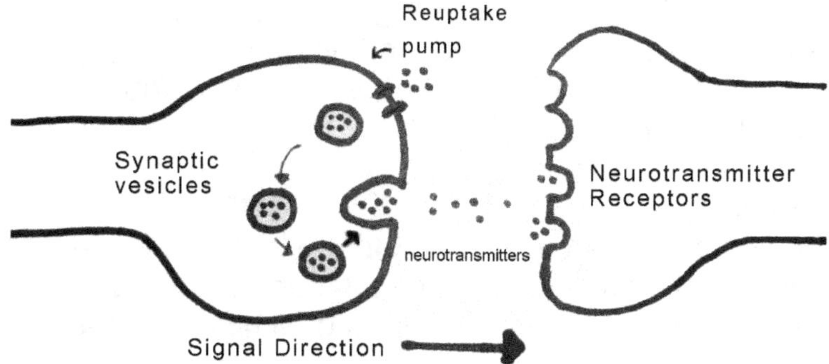

Synapses are an important subject for understanding how drugs work since many conditions can be improved by interacting with this area.

1.6 Drug Dynamic inside the human body

How much a drug is needed to be taken in order to have a therapeutic effect? In reality, everyone will be varied since if you measure a group of people who took the same amount of drug, the concentration of the drug in the blood will be dramatically varied for everyone at the same they measured. So if too little drug remains in the blood, it never reach to desire therapeutic level, but if it's too much, a toxic effect will be resulted. By using a method called Therapeutic Drug Monitoring or TDM, a suitable dosage of drug can be found. There are many factors to cause this variation.

There are four major reasons to be considered.

1. Absorption by Diffusion
Drug molecules can be traveled from high concentration to low concentration without exerting energy. [It's like getting water from the rain, there is no energy required.]

2. Absorption by Active Transport
Drug molecules can be traveled actively with a carrier or a transporter which requires energy. Molecules such as vitamins, bile salt are traveled in this method. [It's like getting water from the water bottle company, you need to pay for that service.]

3. Distribution
Drug molecules can enter into blood stream and distribute to whole body through blood circulation. [Blood vessels are like our freeway system carrying all kinds of stuffs.]

4. Degradation
Drug molecules can be degraded or destroyed by many methods, such as dissolve in water, or with a pH level change, temperature change, or by certain enzymes and also depends on the stability of the drug molecule itself

since it is possible to degrade on its own. [What we used may end up in trash bin and some got recycled.]

One of main ways to expel drug is through kidney.

FYI: Heavy smokers have less theophylline (drug for asthma) concentration in their blood than non-smokers since liver in a heavy smoker will secret more metabolism enzymes to decompose theophylline and thus lower the theophylline concentration in the blood.

Ref: "*Does a One-Size Drug Dose Fit All? Or, Why All the Variability in the Theophylline Blood Concentrations?*" By Kathleen Boje
http://ublib.buffalo.edu/libraries/projects/cases/drug_dosing/drug_dosing_notes.html

1.7 The Effects of Mixing Drugs

Depending on the illnesses, only a few treatments require a single drug, and most of time, multiple drugs are consumed within a day. As more drugs are involved, the probability of having side effects increases a lot more and not proportionally compared to just taking one drug.

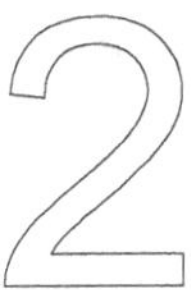

Drugs that are Easy to Understand

2.1 Anti-diarrhea

The symptom of diarrhea is an abnormal condition in the body which results a fast bowel movement in the intestine where additional water is entering into the intestine cell wall as a way to flush the content of intestine out from the body. This is actually a defense mechanism for the intestine. Therefore, by stopping the diarrhea symptom is not a cure for illness since many conditions needed to be considered.

1. Stabilizing the digestive tracks
In case you do not know about what other substances are in the intestine, it has a variety of bacteria that keep you healthy and aid in digestion. These bacteria can keep the digestive track in optimal pH level and inhibit the growth of other harmful bacteria.

Probiotics or good microorganisms live inside the gastrointestinal tracts: Bifidobacterium, Clostridium, Lactic acid bacteria

2. Bowel Movement Inhibitor
Drug such as loperamide hydrochloride can slow down the over stimulated movement in the intestine by combining the protein around the intestine's lining and consequently, it will precipitate out and reduce the water flow and slow down the bowel movement.

3. Anti-inflammatory
When inflammation occurred in the intestinal cells, it will induce diarrhea symptom. Drug such as bismuth can effectively combining with protein to form a water-insoluble area to insulate the inflamed intestinal cells.

4. Absorption
Excessive gases produced in the intestine or over water absorption can increase bowel movement and result in

diarrhea. Drug such as aluminum silicate can effectively absorb excessive water, and while drug like dimethicone is able to reduce excessive gases build up by decrease the surface tension.

5. Bile Salt Sequestrants

After the removal of gallbladder, patients usually developed diarrhea because of the excess bile salt is entering the colon instead of being absorbed by the small intestine. Bile salt or bile acid sequestrants work by inactive bile salt by forming an insoluble complex so less water will enter to the colon and diarrhea can be stopped as a result. An example of drugs is cholestyramine.

6. Analgesics

Drug such as codeine phosphate, can stop diarrhea since block the nerve transmission from the parasympathetic nerve system to intestine. This is a strongest medication for stopping diarrhea.

7. Anticholinergics

Many internal organs are controlled by both sympathetic and parasympathetic nervous system. When over excited parasympathetic nerve system, it will induce diarrhea problem. The scopolamine found in scopolia has an anticholinergics effect where it can slow down the bowel movement by blocking the muscarinic acetylcholine receptors as an antagonist. As a result, muscular contractions become less frequent.

2.2 Gastrointestinal Stimulant - Relieve constipation

Constipation discomfort varies in degrees among people. The main reasons are due to over water absorption from the GI tract or movement in GI track is too slow. It is important to identify what cause the constipation if possible if one experiences chronic symptom. Laxative is usually given for relieving constipation problem if needed. There are four major types of laxatives that act by diffusion method.

1. Osmotic agents and saline laxatives
This type of drugs causes water to enter the intestinal tract and creating pressure to cause muscle contraction. However, loss of electrolytes or dehydration will be resulted as one of side effects. Examples are magnesium oxide, magnesium sulfate, sodium sulfate, magnesium citrate.

2. Fiber products / bulk-forming agents
Substances like psyllium have the effect of increasing the interior volume of the intestinal tract, and this facilitates the bowel movement. In addition, it should be required to be taken along with at least a full glass of water with this type of laxative since it has ability to retain water molecules. Examples are carmellose sodium, guar gum, Psyllium, Metamucil, Methylcellulose, Citrucel.

3. Stool softeners and lubricants
This type of laxative will allow fluids to mix into the stool by increases its surface tension and it will make easier to pass. An example is dioctyl sodium sulfosuccinate (DSS).

4. Carbohydrate Laxative
Drug such as Sorbitol is often a choice for elderly patient who has a weaker liver. It works in similar fashion as the saline laxatives and also it will induce gas forming inside

the GI tract. As a result, it will improve the bowel movement.

Laxatives that work by Simulation

1. Stimulant laxatives work by chemically stimulate the movement of intestinal tract either act on small intestine or large intestine.
For example, Ricinus Communis Oil (Castor oil) acts on small intestine, and bisacodyl or sodium picosulfate works on large intestine. There are many herbal extracts also working at this level.

2. Stimulant laxative like pantethine (a derivative of Vitamin B5) acts on central nervous system to increase bowel movement.

2.3 Anti-gout Medication

Gout is a painful condition which caused by excessive build up of uric acid and leads to crystallize and deposits in joints, tendons, and other tissues and then causes inflammation.
The build up of uric acid was caused by the abnormal nucleotide (purine) metabolism. Purine is one type of the components which make up the DNA.

Purines → hypoxanthine → xanthine → uric acid → uric crystals → Pain

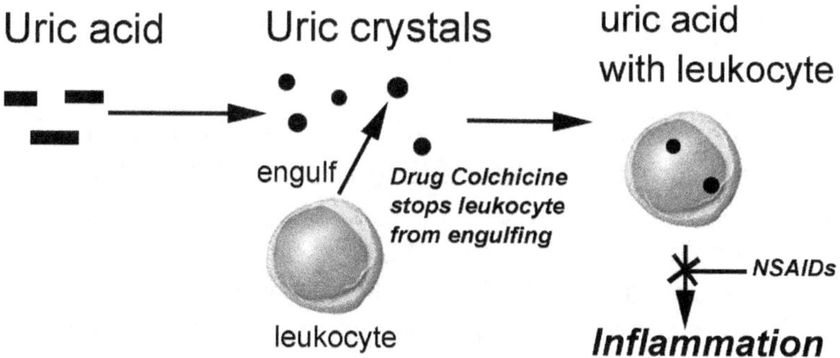

Gout is a recurring medical problem. We can group the drug types by its conditions.

Drugs that Prevent Gout from recurring

In order to control the level of uric acid from building up, drugs like allopurinol, are used to exhaust the enzyme, xanthine oxidase, which creating uric acid from xanthine. As a result, less uric acid will be produced.

Other drugs like probenecid can block kidney's function of recycling the uric acid back to blood stream. As a result, the uric acid is being expelling out more and then the level of uric acid in blood will be dropped. However, urine will be more acidic due to higher concentration of uric acid in the kidney. This will cause stone been forming in the tubes in the kidney. In order to prevent this from happening, drugs like sodium hydrogen carbonate or sodium citrate may be used.

Drugs that Treat Acute Gout Condition or Gout Attack

Colchicine is usually used to treat gout since it has anti-inflammatory effect. Inflammation in gout can be caused by the white blood cells, leukocytes, engulf the deposited crystals. At this stage, the pain in gout is even more since leukocytes usually release lysosomal enzymes and affect the surrounding tissue to cause inflammation. Colchicine works by inhibiting the leukocytes movement by affecting its microtubules.

Drugs like naproxen or indomethacin are all non-steroidal anti-inflammatory drugs (NSAIDs) that can treat pain or inflammation caused by out or other problems such as arthritis, tendonitis. This type of drugs works by blocking the enzyme in your body that makes prostaglandins, which will help to reduce the pain and selling associated with gout.

2.4 Blood-fat Reducers (Antihyperlipidemics Drugs)

The high concentration of fats in the blood is the major cause for blood related illnesses, such as strokes and heart attack. Fats are an essential component in the body. It provides structural framework as you can find it in the cell membrane or on the skin. Fats also make hormones and can be used as an energy source. Unlike carbohydrates or protein that readily used up by the body as source of energy, if body needs to use fat for energy, it must exert a lot of energy to metabolize it. As a result, it is a good material for structure and storage. However, because of its nature of being difficult to be used, it becomes a big problem if the concentration of fat increases in the blood stream. As fat is building up in the blood stream, it tends to stick to the wall and form blockage or decrease the flexibility of the blood vessel. Consequently, this will lead to a serious of dangerous medical problems such as heart attack where heart cannot receive oxygen due to the blockage of its blood supply. For stroke, as the blood vessel loses its flexibility and hardens in its wall, the blood vessel will burst as pressure accumulated and blood clot will be resulted when blood cells flow out of the vessel.

There are many types of fats in the blood we must learn in order to understand how drugs work.

1. Cholesterol

Cholesterol is a popular word nowadays, but do you know it plays important roles in the body. Cholesterol is actually a precursor of many important components in the body, such as hormones, bile acid, and many fat-soluble vitamins.

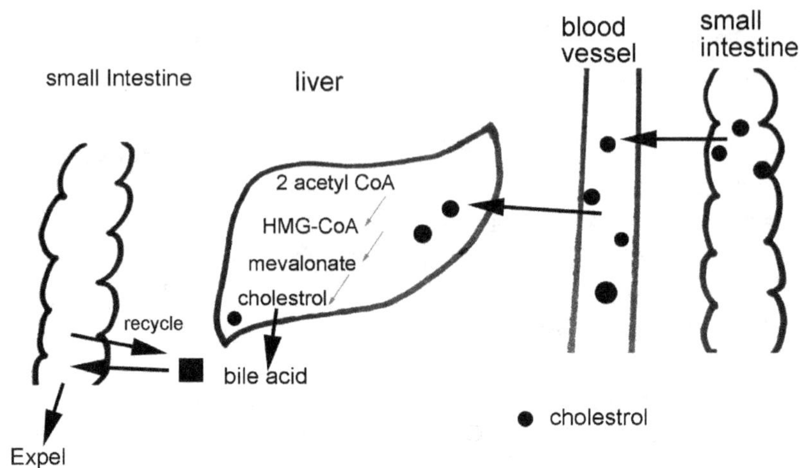

2. Lipoproteins

As we know that fat is not soluble in water and it will be difficult to travel in the water-based bloodstream. Thanks to the lipoprotein, cholesterol and other fat molecules can travel in the blood stream via lipoprotein as its vehicle. In addition, lipoprotein is sophisticated enough to equipped with cell-targeting signal and knows where to go, and just like a GPS. In addition, there are many types of lipoproteins, and you can think them as different buses with different number since they have specific routes and endpoints to travel. In order of increased density, chylomicron is very-low-density lipoprotein (VLDL), and then intermediate-density lipoprotein (IDL), low-density lipoprotein (LDL), and high-density lipoprotein (HDL) is the most dense one. The bus or lipoprotein that has a higher capacity for cholesterol is the one with less density. In fact, LDL is the major carrier of cholesterol in the blood. It can contain approximately 1,500 molecules of cholesterol. We should call it as a ship, not a bus. Isn't it?

3. Triglyceride (TG)

Triglyceride is a major component of chylomicrons and very low density lipoprotein (VLDL). It has a structure consisting of a glyceride plus the fatty acids, and when the

body needs energy, one way is to use TG to get the fatty acid and convert into energy.
Usually people who have higher TG tend to have higher level of LDL (bad cholesterol) and low HDL (good cholesterol). This is a good indicator to tell who is at risk of having a high cholesterol level.

Good cholesterol and Bad cholesterol
Why one is better than the other you may ask? Actually, it is really depending on the route that the carrier is taking. For example, one carrier brings the excess cholesterol away from the blood stream and back to liver, we will call it a good carrier. In this case, it's HDL (not DHL carrier! [This helps you to remember]). On the other hand, VLDL transports TG from the liver to other tissues via bloodstream, which will increase the cholesterol concentration in blood. LDL transports cholesterol throughout the body. In addition, LDL tends to deposit its cholesterol molecules in the inner walls of the arteries that feed the heart and brain. You may think that LDL carries too many packages at one time, and a lot of loosing packages all over the place. Thus, LDL is bad.

After understanding how each component plays a part in the bloodstream, it will be easy to understand how different types of drugs act.

1. Anti HMG-CoA reductase Drugs
HMG-CoA reductase is an enzyme that converts HMG-CoA into mevalonate, a cholesterol precursor. This type of drugs will inhibit the conversion, and it will cause the production of cholesterol to decrease in liver. Since the cholesterol in the liver becomes less, more LDL receptors will be made in order to grab the cholesterol molecules from the blood stream. Consequently, the level of cholesterol will be decreased in the body.
Examples are pravastatin sodium, simvastatin, fluvastatin sodium, atorvastain calcium hydrate (Liptor), pitavastatin calcium, rosuvastatin calcium.

2. Bile acid sequestrants or Ion Exchange Resins
You may know that bile acid is made from cholesterol, and after bile acid aids digestion in the intestinal tract and most of them will be recycled back via bloodstream by the liver. The recycling process is called the enterohepatic circulation where drugs like Colestilan and colestyramine (see section 2.1.5) disrupt the recycling process by sequestering them (using ion exchange method*) in the GI** tract since after forming an insoluble complex that cannot be reabsorbed into bloodstream. As a result, it will decrease cholesterol levels, particular for the LDL since liver will demand more cholesterol by increasing LDL receptors.

*Ion exchange means that it can exchange its chloride anions with anionic bile acids to form a strong bonding complex
**Gastrointestinal tract

3. Probucol
This drug treats coronary artery disease by preventing clogging caused by cholesterol. The reason for cholesterol to cause clogging in the wall of blood vessels is because that the cholesterol molecules in LDL tend to be oxidized and form plaques around the inner wall of blood vessels. Probucol acts to inhibit the oxidation process.

4. Prevent the absorption of Cholesterol from intestinal tract
Drugs like ezetimibe can lower cholesterol levels by preventing cholesterol had been absorbed in the intestine via cholesterol transporter. Cholesterol will be expelled out from the body.

5. Controlling the level of Triglycerides (TG)

Fibrate Type:
Drugs like clofibrate directly lower the level of TG and can promote the conversion of VLDL to LDL and also increase

the level of HDL as well. Examples are clinofibrate, bezafibrate, fenofibrate, and clofibrate.

Nicotinic Acid

Drugs like tocopherol nicotinate, nicomol, niceritrol, decreases synthesis of VLDL and this may decrease TG. In addition, it has shown to raise the HDL level.

Ref: *Influence of nicotinic acid on metabolism of cholesterol and triglycerides in man*
http://www.jlr.org/cgi/content/abstract/22/1/24

2.5 Antiglaucoma Treatment

Aqueous humor is the fluid that circulates inside the eyes. It provides nutrients to the lens and cornea, and also maintains the inner pressure of eye ball in order to keep the shape of the eye ball. In addition, aqueous humor is produced by the epithelia cells of the ciliary body, and it is drain from posterior chamber to anterior chamber and then drain through the canals of Schlemm as it exits the eye. This is known as the primary route aqueous humor flow. The secondary route is via the uveoscleral drainage. Glaucoma is often caused by excessive aqueous humor which lead to high intraocular pressure and it can then damage the optic nerve. There are two types of glaucoma: open angle (chronic) and closed angle (acute).

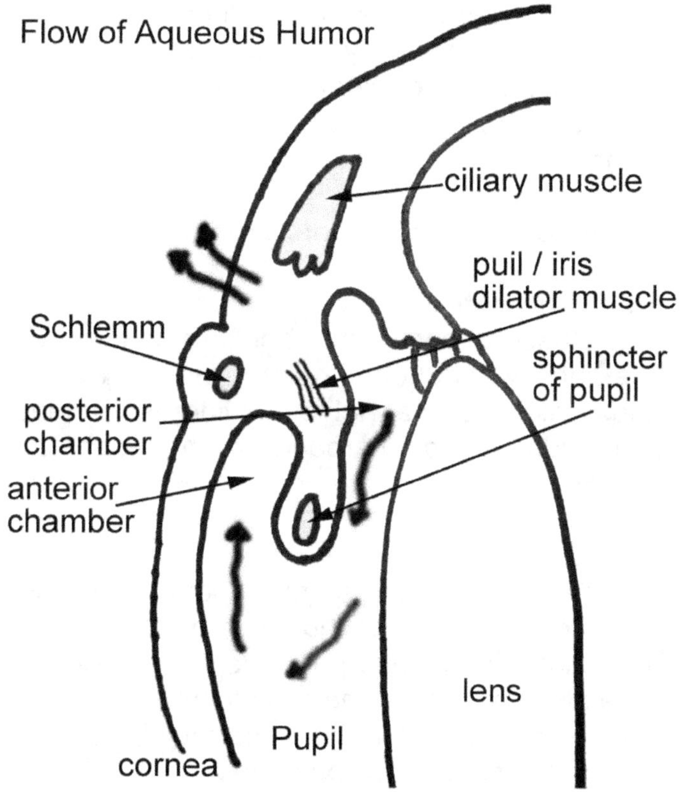

FYI: Normal intraocular pressure is between 10 to 21 mm Hg, and the average is about 16.

Immediate Treatment for Acute angle closure glaucoma (AACG)

1. Highly Diffusible Pressure Reducer

Drugs like D-mannitol, isosorbide, and glycerine, can immediately penetrate eyes and remove water from blood vessels, and reduce water from eye ball and also inhibits the production of aqueous humor from the ciliary body.

2. Carbonic Anhydrase Inhibitors

These drugs work by decreasing the production of aqueous humor since ciliary body will use carbonic anhydrase, an enzyme, to convert carbonic $HCO3^-$ to produce aqueous humor. Examples are acetazolamide, Neptazane, and Daranide.

Other Glaucoma Drugs for Chronic Treatment

1. Parasympathomimetics
These drugs are used to control intraocular pressure by increasing the outflow of aqueous humor from the eye via expanding the Schlemmn channel to be wider. Examples are pilocarpine hydrochloride, carbachol, echothiophate and demecarium.

2. Beta-blockers
The beta-blockers are usually used for hypertension illness since it will reduce heart rate. Using these drugs in eye drops can reduce the intraocular pressure since beta receptors were also involved in the production of aqueous humor. Examples are timolol maleate, carteolol hydrochloride, and betaxolol hydrochloride.

3. Sympathomimetics

Drug like dipivefrin hydrochloride is an epinephrine precursor (or prodrug of epinephrine) that works by decreasing the production of aqueous humor production and increasing outflow of the fluid from the eyes.

4. Prostaglandin

Drug like isopropyl unoprostone, is a prostaglandin analogue which has a similar structure as prostaglandin. It works by increasing the outflow of aqueous humor via the channel of Schlemm and secondary route via the uveoscleral drainage.

5. Optic Nerve Protector

Finally, there is a new class of drug that is still under investigation is to protect the optic nerve. For example, the drug called Namenda (memantine) is waiting for possible approval from FDA where it has shown to prevent shrinkage of visual nerve cells in patients with glaucoma.

The popular herb that is readily available from the counter is gingko biloba, which was reported in "*Ophthalmology*" demonstrate that it can improve the visual field to be wider. The active ingredients, terpenoids and flavonoids may be responsible for improving circulation and its antioxidant properties help preventing free radical damages in the optic nerve.

Ref: http://www.allaboutvision.com/conditions/glaucoma-3-treatment.htm

2.6 Medication for Cataract

A cataract is a clouding of the eye's natural lens. It is commonly caused by chemical changes within the lens of the eye and it is thought to be part of the aging process. However, there is no conclusive explanation of what really causes cataract. Some drugs have side effects of causing cataract as well. Some diabetes is possible to develop cataract as we will discuss it in 3.1.5.

There are two major theories explaining the causes of cataract:

1. Free radical theory.
Ultraviolet, ion irradiation, toxic substances, free radicals can cause cloudy crystal protein denaturation (change its structure) caused by cataracts.

Glutathione is a super antioxidant also found in the lens of the eyes to help protect the lens from damage.

2. Couinaud theory
When the ability of degrading the soluble proteins in the eye become weaker, some amino acids will become so called the Couinaud substance, and it will combine with the lens protein to form cloudy substance and affect the opacity of the lens.

Drug called pirenoxine* believed to bind the soluble protein and prevent the formation of Couinaud substance, and thus, it decreases the chance of formation of the cloudy substance.

* Used in Japan for cataract patients

Some researches have done on using salivary glands hormone to inhibit aging in eye lens since it can lower the calcium concentration in blood vessels and this may reduce the calcium from building up in the lens. Thus, it will prevent cataract from forming.

Please also note that long term use of cortical steroids or some specific drugs will also induce cataract problem.

2.7 Non-Steroidal Anti-inflammatory Drugs (NSAIDs)

Almost all the pain, fever, and inflammation are all related to prostaglandin since it is a potent mediator.

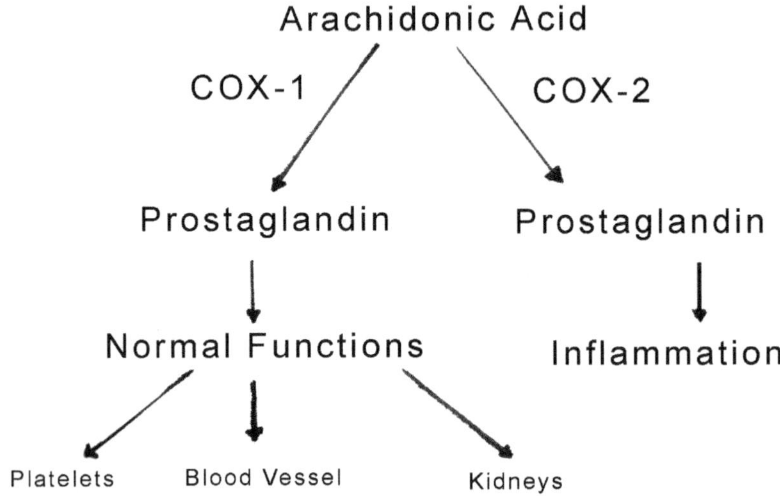

1. Pain
Most of the pains involve with Bradykinin*, but in the presence of prostaglandin, the pain will increase the degree of pain.

*Bradykinin is a protein that involves in inducing vasodilatation (widening blood vessels) and cause smooth muscle to contract and induce pain.

2. Fever
The hypothalamus in the brain regulates the temperature in the body. Prostaglandin can influence hypothalamus directly by setting the temperature higher than normal. Therefore, if the presence of prostaglandin has increased in the blood vessels, fever will be resulted.

3. Inflammation
Prostaglandin can increase the permeability of the blood vessels and cause swelling and inflammation as fluid and plasma protein leak out into the tissue.

A good example of NSAIDs is aspirin or acetylsalicylic acid. Aspirin works by inhibiting the synthesis of prostaglandin from arachidonic acid by cyclooxygenase (COX). In addition, there are two forms of COX. COX-1 carries out the normal, physiological production of prostaglandins, and COX-2 is induced by the inflammatory cells, and is responsible for the prostaglandins that cause inflammation. Therefore, these types of drugs will also have side effect on digestion discomfort since they also targeted the COX-2 and affect the normal digestion process mediate by prostaglandins. Researchers are working hard to find and develop drugs target the COX-2 specifically in order avoid a more serious side effects of stomach lesions and renal toxicity.

Examples of NSAIDs are acetylsalicylic acid (aspirin), meloxicam, mofezolac, etodolac, nabumetone, sulindac, diclofenac, azltoprofen, mefenamic acid, and tiaramide.

2.8 Treating Prostate Enlargement

As the prostate becomes enlarged, the urethra becomes narrow. Urine flows from the bladder through the urethra will become more difficult and require more pressure and energy to push out urine out of body. Either shrinking the prostate or making the urethra wider will help this condition. By the age of 70s, almost 70% of men have some degrees of prostate enlargement problem.

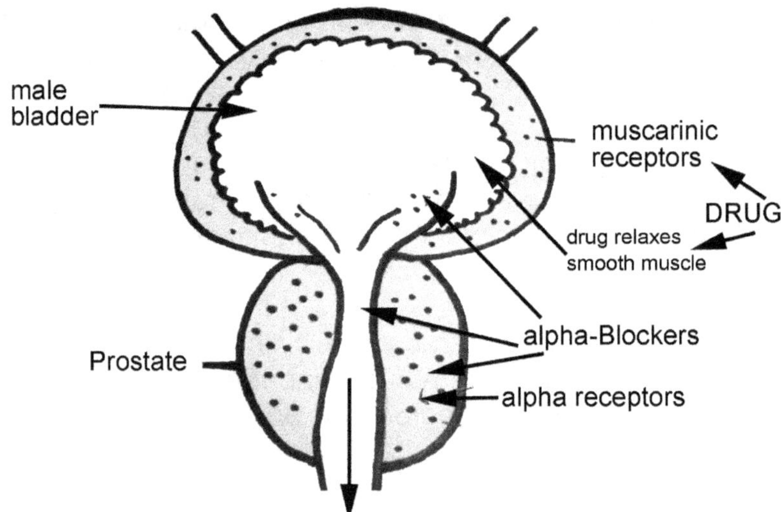

Symptoms of enlarged prostate can include:

- A weak or slow urinary stream
- A feeling of incomplete bladder emptying
- Difficulty starting urination
- Urgency to urinate
- Frequent urination

There are three major types of drugs that improve the prostate enlargement condition.

Prostate Inhibitor

The prostate gland continues to grow in a man's life in a phase fashion, but only until older age like 50s, it increases its growth rate. This is due to the sex hormone imbalance with aging. Men produce both the male hormone testosterone and female hormone estrogen that circulating in the body. But until ages, the production of estrogen does not slow down but instead, it continues to increase. Finally, it causes an imbalance compared to the concentration of testosterone. As the relative level of testosterone decreases, the testosterone receptors on the prostate will increase in order to obtain more testosterone. Consequently, this will cause the cells on the prostate gland to proliferate and grow. In detail, the prostate gland development requires testosterone to convert into dihydrotestosterone (DHT) by 5-alpha reductase.

Examples are chlormadione acetate, allylestrenol.

Alpha Blocker Drugs
These drugs are blocking alpha receptors on cells of urethra and bladder and prevent the contraction of smooth muscle that main caused the difficulty of urination. As a result, it will widen the urethra and improve urination.

Examples are tamsulosin, naftopidil.

Improvement on frequent urination condition
Frequent urination is caused by the reduced capacity of bladder to hold urine. Drugs like the flavoxate hydrochloride increase the bladder by relaxing the smooth muscle cells of the bladder wall.

Similarly over stimulation on the bladder will cause it to have the urgency to urinate. Tolterodine tartrate is a drug that works by blocking the nerve impulse that tells the bladder to contract. Since this type of drug is actually a muscarinic receptor antagonist, which meansthat it works by competing against acetylcholine for the acetylcholine receptor. Acetylcholine is the natural neurotransmitter that supposes to relay the signal in the synapse area if it binds to acetylcholine receptor. (See Section 1.5 for Synapses)

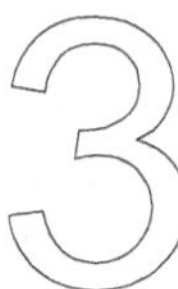

Drugs that are Understandable if you have a little more time!

If you have read up to this point, you should have a pretty idea on how drugs work. Let us explore a little more on this subject and discover what other drugs are there to treat those commonly known illnesses.

3.1 Medication for Diabetes

Diabetes or known as diabetes mellitus is an abnormal condition where utilization of glucose, the main source of energy, becomes the problem in the body. As a result, this leads to various complications such as loss sight and vision, discomfort in kidney, and affecting the nervous system. As you may have heard insulin before, it is a hormone produced by pancreas that enables cells to absorb glucose. Cells use glucose to turn into energy in the format of ATP.

So diabetes can cause by either when the pancreas does not produce insulin enough (This is called Diabetes Type 1) or when the cells do not respond to insulin properly (This is called Diabetes Type 2). There are other forms of diabetes such as for some pregnant women (about 2%), they may suffer gestational diabetes because either some hormones block the normal action of insulin or body of mother just cannot meet the extra demand for insulin. As a result, blood sugar will be high.

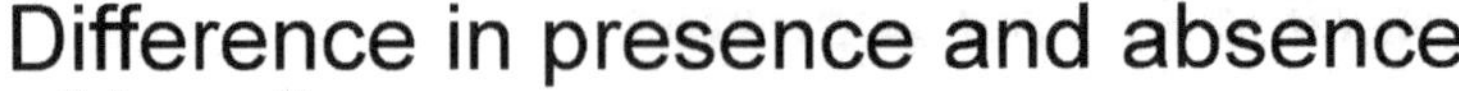

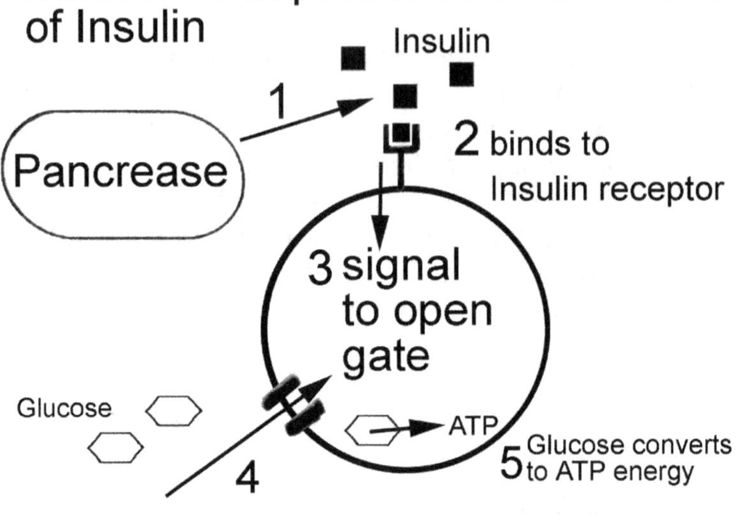

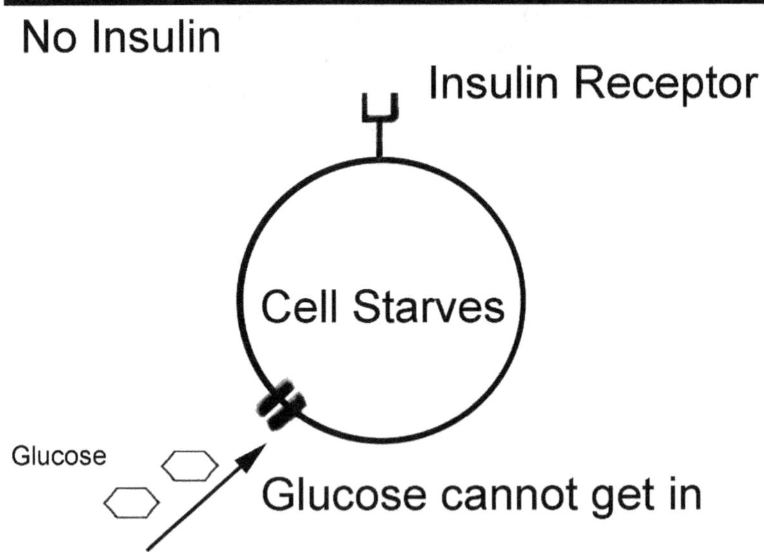

Here are different types of anti-diabetic drugs:

1. Oral Medication

The sulfonylurea (SU) has been available for many years and it works by increasing the secretion of insulin from the pancreas via acting on the pancreatic beta cells. Examples are tolbutamide, glibenclamide, and nateglinide.

2. Biguanides

This drug does not have as strong effect as the SU to induce beta cells to secrete insulin. Nevertheless, it helps by reducing the production of glucose from the liver, and inhibits the intestines from absorbing glucose. In addition, it also help other cells especially the skeletal muscle to uptake glucose. Overall, it decreases the level of glucose in the blood. Examples are buformin and metformin.

3. Insulin-Sensitizing Drugs

In some cases, the level of insulin is not abnormally low and it seems like that the glucose in the blood still not be regulated well and remains at high level. This is called the Insulin Resistance condition. This happens mostly at obese people and overeaten without enough exercise. The drug thiazolidinediones (TZDs) can help cells to better respond to insulin. It acts by activating PPAR-γ* and decreasing TNF-α** in the fat cells or adipocytes.

* PPAR-γ is **p**eroxisome **p**roliferators **a**ctivated-gamma **r**eceptor. It is a transcription factor that has shown to improve insulin sensitivity.
** TNF-α is Tumor Necrosis Factor-alpha that inhibits the insulin receptor.

4. α-Glucosidase Inhibitors
This drug is used for Type 2 condition and works by blocking carbohydrates from digestion in the intestine and thus it lowers the blood sugar. Since it works by competing for binding the enzyme needed to digest carbohydrate, it is more practical to take this drug before the meal. An example is acarbose.

5. Aldose Reductase Inhibitor

Aldose reductase is an enzyme converts glucose to sorbitol*. For unknown reason that as in some diabetes, the body becomes poor management for glucose when patients had diabetic problem after many years. The body tends to convert excessive glucose into sorbitol for storage. However, the excessive level of sorbitol will lead to swelling in tissue and induce nerve damage (Schwann cells of the nervous system) in the body or diabetic neuropathy. In fact, this also leads to the development of the lens cataracts. The drug, epalrestat, is an aldose reductase inhibitor that has shown to delay the progression of neuropathy.

*Sorbitol or sorbit, a type of sugar, is found naturally in a wide range of fruits and plants. Our body also produces sorbitol from glucose since it will convert into fructose in a later step. Fructose is used as a source of energy for some specific cells, such as sperm cells and some liver cells.

6. Injectable Insulin

Injecting insulin directly to the body helps the Type 1 diabetes since the body is no longer produce the insulin hormone. You can think insulin is like a flag that once it's bind to an insulin receptor, components related to glucose metabolism will see that flag as a sign to uptake glucose by transporting glucose into the cell. Without that flagging signal, the cells are literally starved even there are plenty of glucose surrounding them. In addition, the liver cells are aware of the blood sugar level from the stimulation of insulin in the blood stream, and will adjust it by storing glucose.

3.2 Medication for Heart Failure

Heart failure is a condition in which the heart is overloading and becomes weaken as it is not able to pump the blood completely. There are chronic and acute types of heart failure. Regardless of which type, the symptoms include difficult in breathing and swollen in lung.

Blocking Angiotensin II signal pathway
will lower blood pressure

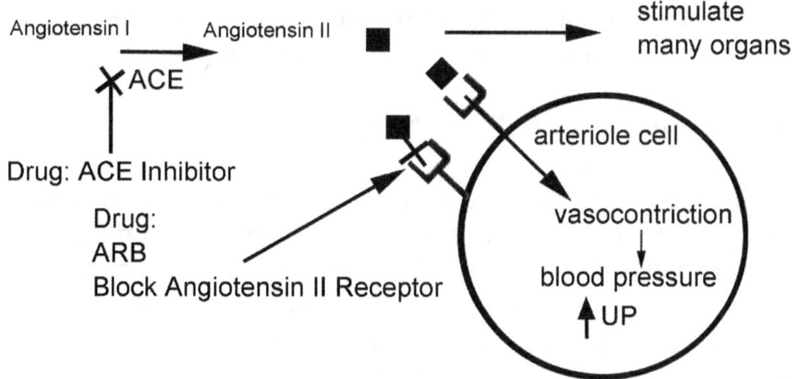

ACE Inhibitors

These drugs are used to inhibit angiotensin-converting enzyme (ACE) and it is the first choice of drug since it can take the load out from the heart and give time to let the heart to recover back to normal. It reduces the volume of blood pumped back to the heart and decrease blood pressure since it widens the blood vessel. Thus, this drug is also used for hypertension patients to lower their blood pressure. The adverse side effect is usually accompanied by a persistent of dry cough which was believed that the drug also increases in bradykinin level. (See 2.7.1) Examples are captopril and enalapril maleate.

Angiotensin II Receptor Blockers (ARB)

These drugs have the same effect as ACE inhibitors, except they are acting on the angiotensin receptors. In contrast, ACE inhibitors are acting on the enzyme which produces angiotensin II. An example of ARB is losartan potassium.

Beta-1 Receptors Stimulants

These drugs like dopamine hydrochloride, stimulates beta-1 receptors in the heart which causes more complete and forceful contraction since more cyclic AMP (c-AMP) is able to induce the contraction of heart muscle cells.

Phosphodiesterase III Inhibitors

For example, milrinone is a phosphodiesterase III inhibitor, which enhances the effect of c-AMP by increasing Ca^{2+}-ATPase activity* on the cardiac sarcoplasmic reticulum. As a result, it enhances the relaxation of left ventricle of heart to increase heart contraction. Examples are milrinone, amrinone, olprinone hydrochloride.

* Ca^{2+}-ATPase activity is an activity made by a transport protein for removing Ca^{2+} ions out from the cell. Since this is a transporter requires energy, the ATP is involving in supplying that energy to this transporter.

A note about using beta-blocker for treating heart failure

It has been thought that patients with heart failure should not take beta blocker since it may weaken the already weak heart. After many researches and clinical trials have been made since 2000, many patients can be benefit by taking beta blocker drugs since it can help the heart to give more rest to recover. However, patients must consult with physician for the suitable beta-blocker drugs for heart failure treatment.

3.3 Medication for Hypertension (High Blood Pressure)

Hypertension is a chronic condition where the pressure of blood vessel remains high. There is no one root cause or specific location for this condition since blood vessels are used by all tissues in the body. It should be looked at it as an overall body condition. Therefore, it is recommended that lifestyle must be changed along with the hypertension treatment in order to really improve this medical condition since it's a chronic problem and there is no fast way to treat it.

Here are the major types of anti-hypertension drugs:

1. Calcium Channel Blockers
Since the smooth muscle cells on the wall of blood vessels can control the width of the blood vessels, either widens or narrows it. In detail, the movement of calcium channel controls the constriction of the muscle cells and when there are more Ca^{2+} ions enter into blood vessels, the muscle will contract and narrow the blood vessels and consequently, the pressure in blood vessels will also rise. Calcium channel blockers can lower blood pressure by blocking calcium ions from entering into the calcium channels.

Examples are amlodipine, aranidipine, and nifedipine.

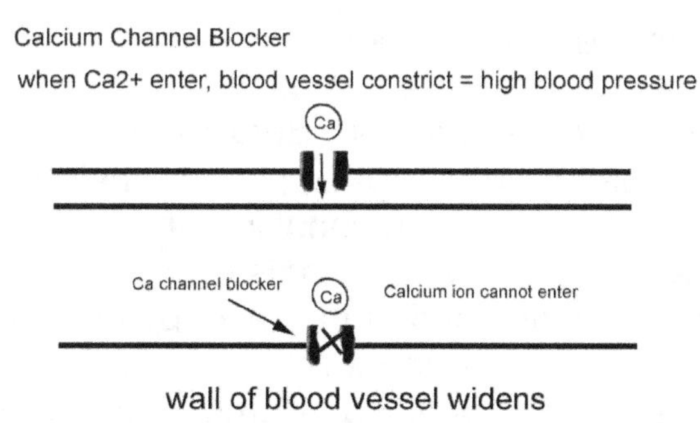

2. Angiotensin-Converting Enzyme (ACE) Inhibitor
We have already covered ACE inhibitor to treat heart failure earlier in Section 3.2. These drugs also can use for treating hypertension since by inhibiting ACE, it blocks the conversion of angiotensin I to angiotensin II so that angiotensin II will not bind to the receptor to induce muscle contraction. Thus, no muscle contraction on the blood vessels means that the diameter of blood vessel remains the same and no pressure will increase in the blood vessels.

Examples are captopril, alacepril, cilazapril, benazepril, and trandolapril.

3. Angiotensin II Receptor Blockers (ARBs)
These drugs were also used for heart failure as discussed in Section 3.2. These drugs act on the angiotensin II receptors by blocking the receptors from angiotensin II. As a result, the smooth muscle cells will not contracted, and this helps to lower blood pressure. In addition, ARBs can bind to one of the two types of receptor, the AT1, and not AT2. Some studies also showed that AT2 can lower blood pressure if it is being stimulated. Examples are losartan, candesartan, and telmisartan.

4. Beta-blockers

These beta receptors are located mainly in the heart and kidneys. Once these receptors are stimulated by epinephrine*, the heart will beat faster. Beta-blockers are the most commonly used drug for treating hypertension that I have heard. For hypertension condition, the main focus is to lower the blood pressure. In this class of drugs, it can help to reduce the work load of the heart by making both the blood vessel and tissue more relax to contain more blood and as a result, less blood returns to the heart. In addition, beta-blockers help slow down the heart rate and it can treat hypertension patients who also have arrhythmias (abnormal heart beat rhythm). Patients taking beta-blocker must also know that sudden withdrawal of beta-blocker can cause adverse effects such as heart attack since it may induce a sudden increase in heart rate and blood pressure. Examples are propranolol, nadolol, pindolol, atenolol, acebutolol, and celiprolol.

*Epinephrine is also known as adrenaline, the hormone secreted by adrenal gland.

5. Diuretics

Another method of lowing blood pressure is commonly used is to get rid of excess water from the blood vessels. This is done by diuretics drugs especially the thiazide-type. These drugs can help the kidneys to get rid of water and salt from the body. It acts on blocking the reabsorption of sodium ions on the distal convoluted tubule in kidney and water will be expelled in the urine. Examples are trichlormethiazide, meticrane, furosemide, and triamteren.

6. Alpha-blockers

In contrast to the beta-receptors located on heart and kidneys, alpha receptors are located on the wall of blood vessels. Normally, alpha receptors are responsible for constricting the blood vessel when they are stimulated. Alpha-blockers act on blocking the receptors and inactivate the receptors' function. Some drugs are more selective in binding only the alpha 1 receptors, which are more effective in helping the blood vessels to be relaxed and more blood are carried and blood pressure are also decreased. Examples of alpha-blockers are prazosin, bunazosin, terazosin, urapidil.

Despite many drugs are effectively controlled blood pressure, there are no actual drugs to cure hypertension for now and patients usually have to take the medication for the rest of their lives. Nevertheless, there are many researches have shown some promising results and evidence that doing non-strenuous exercises such as Tai Chi* or Falun Gong** can have beneficial effect on hypertension problem.

*Studies conducted by the Johns Hopkins University School of Medicine
http://findarticles.com/p/articles/mi_m0675/is_4_20/ai_90924135/

**Studies done by Dr.Lili Feng at Baylor College of Medicine in Texas

3.4 Peptic Ulcer Treatment

Peptic ulcer is an ulcer occurring in an area of gastrointestinal (GI) tract. It is usually acidic and very painful symptom. The erosion of GI wall is not only painful, but also can lead to complication such as internal bleeding. Most of peptic ulcer is caused by bacteria called *Helicobacter pylori* which indirectly increase the production of gastrin, which stimulates the production of gastric acid. Consequently, this will lead to erosion. Another cause may be come from the use of NSAIDs drugs. (See 2.7.3)

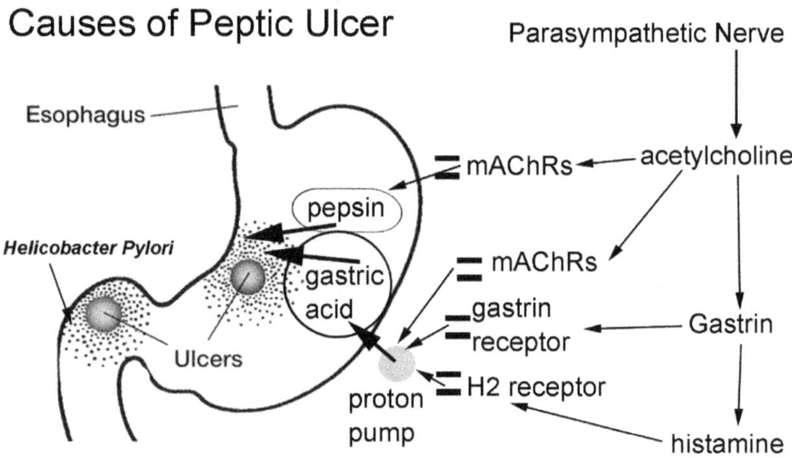

Here are the major treatments for peptic ulcer:

1. Antibiotics

Since *Helicobacter pylori* cannot survive in any acidic level lower than pH 4, *Helicobacter pylori* produces great amount of urease enzyme that can produce ammonia and eventually neutralizes gastric acid by surrounding bicarbonate. As a result, colonization of *Helicobacter pylori* in the stomach will cause chronic ulcer problem. Many antibiotics such as omeprazole and amoxicillin have been used together to eradicate it. However, there are some bacteria that are antibiotic-resistant. Examples of drugs are amoxicillin and clarithromycin.

2. Reducing Acidity Drugs

The membrane lining in the digestive system normally stands up the strong acidic pH1 ~ pH2 gastric acid. But with the infection from *Helicobacter pylori* or under stress, the mucous membrane will reduce its ability to counteract the acidic environment. So in order to prevent the wound mucous membrane from getting worse, reducing the acidity can promote healing of the damaged cells.

1. H2 Blockers (Histamine H2 Antagonist)

The mast cells are generated in bone marrow and present in the blood vessels and most tissues. It produces histamine where it mediates both allergic reaction and digestive acid production in the stomach. Thus there are two types of histamine receptor where, H1 receptors relate to allergic pathway, and H2 receptors relate to digestion. One of these drugs acts as antagonist where it binds to the H2 receptor and decreases the production of acid in the stomach. Examples are cimetidine, famotidine, and nizatidine.

2. Gastrin Inhibitors

The gastrin enzyme will stimulate the inner wall of stomach to secrete acid and promote the process of histamine to bind H2 receptor. Thus, these gastrin inhibitors will inhibit or decrease the acidic production for digestion. An example is proglumide.

3. Muscarinic receptors (mAChRs) Inhibitors

The neurotransmitters we learned previously in nerve cells about how signals are transmitted in the synapses also played an important role in digestion since acetylcholine will stimulate the production of histamine for increasing the secretion of gastric acid in the stomach. Clinically, these drugs can reduce the pain and the problems associated with ulcer. Copolamine butylbromide is an example of these drugs.

4. Proton Pump Inhibitors (PPIs)

These drugs are the most potent and long-lasting effect compared to the previous drugs since all those three ways of digestions will end up to proton pump as the last step of producing the gastric acid. So by applying these drugs like benzimidazole, it will inhibit the gastric acid production very effectively. However, these drugs will weaken the defense mechanism against potential harmful organisms that commonly are destroyed in the strong acidic stomach.

5. Antacids

By taking antacids, it effectively neutralizes the gastric acid in the stomach in order to prevent the further erosion to the ulcer stomach. A good example is dried aluminum hydroxide gel, where it's a weaker base. In contrast, whereas using a strong base substance will induce more gastric acid.

3. Strengthen Stomach Drugs

Once the wall of stomach has been damaged, it becomes a necessity to find ways to heal and alleviate stomach from more damages from the acid. Here are drugs that actively strengthen and protect stomach in this period.

1. Sucralfate

This drug can bind hydrochloric acid in the stomach to form viscous film around the wall of stomach. It then acts as a protector or an acid buffer so that acid is not penetrating to the damage wall. This drug should be taken before a meal in order to be effective.

2. Aldioxa
This drug is also known as the membrane repair agent for the stomach since it can promote the repair of stomach cell wall.

3. Teprenone
This drug is used in Japan* as a gastric mucosal protective drug since it induces the production of gastric mucosa and mucosa is very effective in insulating acid from the wall.

*http://content.karger.com/ProdukteDB/produkte.asp?Doi=201310

4. Cetraxate Hydrochloride
This drug promotes the production of gastric mucosa.

5. Prostaglandin

Drugs like enprostil is a synthetic prostaglandin that resembles prostaglandin E2 that can prevent and treat peptic ulcers since prostaglandin can prevent gastric HCl secretion. It is also involved in process of cytoprotection in the deep mucosa. The mechanism of cytoprotection is not well known yet, but it shows that prostaglandin E can increase gastric mucosal blood flow (GMBF) and this leads to cell protection.

Ref:
http://www.ncbi.nlm.nih.gov/pubmed/9359921
http://grande.nal.usda.gov/ibids/index.php?mode2=detail&origin=ibids_references&therow=121332

3.5 Osteoporosis Treatment

Calcium plays various vital roles in the body in the areas of lung's gas exchange, bone development, digestive system and the nerve system. Bone serves as the storage for calcium. When body needs calcium, calcium will flow into blood vessels in the process called bone resorption, which is mediated by osteoclast cells. The opposite process is called ossification (mediated by osteoblast cells) where bone is formed and calcium is deposited and store inside. In order to keep bone healthy, body implement a process of bone remodeling where bone is constantly in bone resorption and ossification process. Osteoporosis is a medical condition where an imbalance in the process of bone remodeling where the rate of ossification is slower than the bone resorption process.

Bone Remodeling

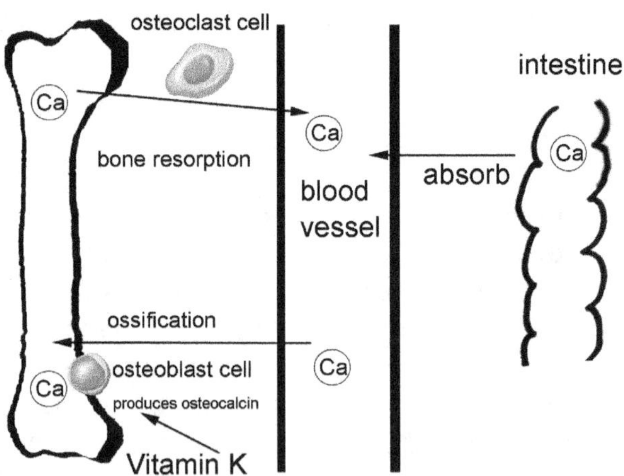

Here are drugs for osteoporosis.

1. Calcium Replenisher

When the concentration of calcium drops in the blood, which is monitored by the parathyroid gland, the osteoclast cells will become more active in removing calcium from bone. In this way, it results in increased calcium concentration the blood. By taking the calcium replenisher, such as calcium gluconate, it increases the calcium concentration and inhibits the activities from osteoclast cells. Examples are calcium gluconate, calcium lactate, and calcium L-aspartate.

2. Active Form of Vitamin D (D3)

Vitamin D3, also known as cholecalciferol, is the form of vitamin D naturally formed in the skin from 7-dehydorcholesterol as a result of UVB radiation from sunlight. It controls absorption of calcium by intestinal cells and also increases the calcium concentration in the blood.

3. Estrogen Replacement

At onset of menopause for women, the decreased production of estrogen often leads to osteoporosis called postmenopausal osteoporosis. Since estrogen also regulates the osteoclast apoptosis*, as estrogen level drops, there are more osteoclast than normal and this leads to more calcium taking away from bone into blood. An example of drugs is estriol.

*Apoptosis can be the last phase of a cell life where a cell is programmed to self-destruct.

4. SERM – Selective Estrogen Modulator

The SERMs drugs are used for treatment of postmenopausal osteoporosis since it activates the estrogen receptors. However, these drugs act the exactly opposite when comparing to estrogen since they do not stimulate uterus and breast tissue like the estrogen. Thus, they only assist at bone formation and this has less possibility of causing breast cancer since they only activated the beta-estrogen receptors and not the alpha receptors. An example of drugs is raloxifene.

5. Antiresorptive Drug

Elcatonin or ECT is known to relieve pain in postmenopausal osteoporosis in women or patients with bone pain. It can suppress the action on bone resorption and promote bone formation. Currently, the substance can be obtained from eel and salmon.

6. Vitamin K

Vitamin K is most popular in playing a role in blood clotting. It also plays an important role in bone formation. Some researches have shown that vitamin K may be necessary for the production of osteocalcin synthesized by osteoblasts, the bone forming cells.

7. Bone Resorption Inhibitors

These drugs are synthetic bisphosphonate analog of the naturally occurring inhibitor of bone formation, pyrophosphate. An example of drugs is etidronate disodium.

8. Ipriflavone

This substance is found abundantly in plants and it is type of bioflavonoid. It works by inhibit bone resorption and mostly it is used to treat postmenopausal osteoporosis by allowing the osteoblasts to increase its bone density.

3.6 Treatments for Thyroid Disease

Thyroid is located in the neck and it controls and regulates the levels of various hormones in the blood and body's metabolism. It produces thyroid hormones T3 and T4, and only T3 is actually being used directly by the cells for specific protein production. T4 enters into cells will then be converted to T3 eventually. Some thyroid diseases are caused by autoimmune disorder. So many drugs developed can only help to regulate the normal thyroid functions and not able to actual treat the diseases if it's autoimmune caused.

***T3** – triiodothyronine
***T4** - thyroxine

Here are the major drugs used to treat thyroid disease.

1. Desiccated Thyroid
Desiccated thyroid is natural substance that has been used over hundred years which contain both T3 and T4 and can use to treat hypothyroidism. Some patients may be allergic to this since it is usually derived from gland of pigs. The concentration of T3 and T4 varies from these sources.

2. Synthetic T4
Levothyroxine is also known as L-thyroxine, and it is a synthetic T4 that can be readily converted into T3 by cells.

3. Synthetic T3
Liothyronine is directly acting on the body to increase metabolic rate and promote body's protein synthesis process.

Treatment for Hyperthyroidism or Overactive Thyroid

1. Thyroperoxidase Inhibitor

Thyroperoxidase is an enzyme used to convert iodine-containing substance to iodine and add iodine to thyroglobulin that eventually leads to the synthesis of thyroxine (T4). Consequently, the drug like thiamazole can inhibit the enzyme and help reducing the concentration of thyroid hormone.

2. Iodine

Iodine is stored in a protein called thyroglobulin, and it is necessary for the synthesis of thyroid hormones, T4 and T3. However, excessive intake of iodine will result in preventing the production of thyroid hormone. In fact, many surgeries treating hyperthyroidism requested patients to take iodine treatment with anti-thyroid drugs in order to lower the levels of thyroid hormones before the operation.

3.7 Medication for Angina Pectoris

Enough oxygen supply and nutrients provided to the heart cells are crucial for the functions of the heart since heart muscles are constantly working. Coronary arteries are the blood vessels supplying to the heart. Thus, once there is a problem with these arteries, it will reduce the heart productivity and may lead to death. Angina Pectoris is the condition when there is not enough oxygen supply to the heart muscle and often accompany with severe chest pain.

There are two major ways to help this condition immediately. One is to increase the oxygen supply to the coronary arteries, and another is reducing the workload of the heart so that the heart muscle does not need to work that hard. As we have discussed in 3.2, those drugs help reduce workload of heart are also used to treat angina pectoris.

Here are the drugs that treat Angina Pectoris.

1. Nitrates
A good example for this group of drugs is nitroglycerin. Nitroglycerin is known for very long time since its application in making explosive in 1800s. This substance is also used as medicine to treat angina since it effectively widens the blood vessels by relaxing the smooth muscles cells in the inner vessel walls. As a result, the capacity of bringing oxygen by the coronary arteries increases and the volume of blood in the heart is reduced. In this way, it helps heart to get more oxygen and less workload at the same time. In detail, nitroglycerin can contribute the production of nitric oxide in the body, and the more nitric oxide there is, the more c-GMP (cyclic guanosine monophospate) will be converted from GTP (cyclic guanosine triphospates). Finally, more c-GMP will trigger the relaxation of heart muscle since the concentration of

Ca^{2+} (calcium) ions is reduced inside the cells. As a result, arteries will be widened.

2. Calcium Channel Blockers
As discussed in 3.3.1, Calcium Channel Blockers can lower blood pressure by blocking calcium ions from entering into the calcium channel. In this way, it will reduce the workload of heart. In addition, some angina conditions are caused by the spasm of the coronary arteries, and Calcium Channel Blockers can help to stabilize it and prevent this from recurring. Examples are nitrendipine, benidipine, nisoldipine, and verapamil.

3. Beta-blockers
As discussed in 3.2 and 3.3.4, beta-blocker can help to slow down the heart rate and thus reducing the workload of heart. Examples are atenolol, carvedilol, and labetalol.

4. Coronary Arterial Vasodilators
These vasodilators can prevent angina from recurring as they acts on widening the blood vessels of heart arteries. For example, Nicorandil works by contributing of making nitric oxide to guanylate cyclase, the enzyme that makes c-GMP. In this way, the concentration of c-GMP quickly induces calcium ions flow and cause both arterial [blood going into the heart] and venous [blood going out from the heart] vasodilatations. Other examples are dipyridamole and dilazep hydrochloride.

3.8 Anti-thrombotic Drugs

Thrombosis is the formation of a blood clot inside the blood vessel. Thrombosis can happen in any blood vessels in the body. Most fatal and commonly seen thromboses are happening in the brain as cerebral thrombosis and in the heart as arterial thrombosis.

Formation of blood clot is a complex process. To simplify it, we have 2 major systems in making the blood clot. One is the platelet plug mechanism and another is the coagulation. In the coagulation system, there is involvement of fibrinogens which is the subsystem inside the complex process.

Here are drugs inhibit the process involved in the platelet plug mechanism.

1. Aspirin (acetylsalicylic acid)
In order to reduce the thromboxane A2 from making the blood clot from platelet, taking aspirin can lower the production of thromboxane A2. In detail, the synthesis of thromboxane A2 is actually assisted by the prostaglandin, and aspirin can inhibit the production of prostaglandin, and indirectly, it prohibits the platelet plug mechanism. However, dosage of aspirin must be carefully administrated since over certain amount of aspirin will reverse its effect and actually aid the platelet plug mechanism instead.

2. Ozagrel Sodium
Ozagrel Sodium can inhibit the production of thromboxane A2 via prohibiting Thromboxane 2 Synthase and also inhibiting the converting of prostaglandin* to thromboxane A2. Since this drug can also inhibit the platelet plug process even in the smaller blood vessels, it is good to treat cerebral thrombosis.

* Prostaglandin is produced in various locations in the body and there are many different forms of it. Particular Prostaglandin I2 or PGI2 (prostacyclin) can inhibit platelet aggregation and widen the blood vessel wall.

3. Ticlopidine

This drug inhibits platelet plug mechanism by changing the platelet membranes so that platelet cannot be further linked with fibrogens and it further increases the concentration off c-AMP which inhibits the production of thromboxane A2. Clinically, this drug shows effective in treating thrombosis.

4. Sarpogrelate hydrochloride

This drug works as a 5-HT2 receptor antagonist, which can inhibit the platelet aggregation. Normally, 5-HT2 receptor is bind by the neurotransmitter serotonin (5-hydroxtryptamine) and has effect on nerve system, but it also plays role in aggregation of platelets.

Here are drugs that inhibit the process involved in the coagulation mechanism.

1. Herparin Sodium

Heparin is a naturally-occurring substance produced by the white blood cells, mainly the basophils and mast cells. It acts as an anticoagulant which can prevent the formation of clots by causing the shape of enzyme, thrombin, to be non-functional and then affects the formation of fibrin from fibrinogen (insoluble strands of fibrin).

2. Warfarin

Vitamin K plays an important role in coagulation since it can be used to produce coagulation factors VII, IX, X and II. This drug effectively inhibits the effects of Vitamin K in the coagulation by preventing Vitamin K being used by the coagulation process.

Here are drugs capable of dissolving the fibrin in the coagulation mechanism.

Fibrin is the final product produced from the coagulation cascade. It is an insoluble protein that forms a mesh that covers the wound site. In contrast, the clot degrading process or also known as fibrinolysis begins with plasminogen converted into plasmin by urokinase and tissue plasminogen activator (t-PA), and finally, plasmin is able to dissolve fibrin blood clots.

1. Urokinase*

This is naturally-occurring substance that promotes the process of converting plasminogen into plasmin. It is better to administrate this drug locally or else it may cause internal bleeding.

*The urokinase was originally discovered in the urine as implied by the name.

2. Tissue Plasminogen Activator (t-PA)

This group of drugs is commonly used in certain patients who have a heart attack or stroke since it is effectively dissolved clot. Examples are alteoplase, tisokinase, monteplase, pamiteplase, and nasaruplase.

3.9 Medications for Migraine

Currently, it is believed that migraine relates to abnormal constriction and widens of blood vessels in the head area and triggers a serious of symptoms including headache. The actual cause of migraine headache is unknown at this time. There are two major theories possible explaining the causes and drugs are developed and implement according to these theories. They are the Platelet Theory and the Trigeminal Nerve Theory.

In Platelet Theory, it is believed that all stimuli such as stress, smell, and sensitive to light, sleepless can activate the platelet mechanism to eventually lead to less serum and vasodilatation causes stimulating the nerve system abnormally.

In Trigeminal Nerve Theory, it is believed that the cause of repetitive pains and headaches occurred in or relate to the Trigeminal Nerve.

Here are the drugs to treat the acute migraine attack.

1. Ergotamine
Since ergotamine shares similar structures with many neurotransmitters such as serotonin, it can act as an agonist to the 5-HT receptor and constriction of blood vessels will be resulted. Another example is dihydroergotamine mesilate.

2. NSAIDs
As discussed in 2.3 and 2.7, NSAIDs prevents the synthesis of prostaglandin by COX-2 and thereby reducing the level of prostaglandin and pain will be reduced. An example is aspirin.

3. Sumatriptan

This drug is a new kind of drug and since it has a similar structure to serotonin (5HT), and it affects the blood vessel to constrict back to normal when it acts as 5-HT 1D agonist. In addition, it shows pain reduction in Trigeminal Nerve since it inhibits the release of Calcitonin gene-related peptide (CGRP)* from Trigeminal ganglion.

* Calcitonin gene-related peptide plays a role in headache.

Here are the drugs to prevent migraine from coming back.

1. Calcium Channel Blockers
As discussed in 3.3.1 and 3.7.2, Calcium Channel Blockers are used to lower blood pressure. For preventing migraine, these drugs should also be helpful in widening the blood vessels. A good example of these drugs is lomerizine hydrochloride. However, this type of drug should not be used during acute migraine attack.

2. Beta-blockers
As discussed in 3.2, 3.3.4 and 3.7.3, beta-blocker is also used in lowering blood pressure. It is also commonly used for preventing migraine since it relaxes blood vessels. An example is propranolol.

3. Antidepressant Drugs
An example of antidepressant drugs used for treating chronic migraine is amitriptyline. It increases the levels of two neurotransmitters in the brain, which are serotonin and norepinephrine*. The effective dosage for this drug varies from patients to patients. Patients need to be cautious when taking this type of drug concurrent with other drugs or herb supplement such as St. John's wort and need to consult with physicians for possible adverse drug interactions with hypericin found in this herb. Since St. John's wort claims to help promote a positive mood, many people use it for antidepressant purpose.

* Norepinephrine has dual roles as a hormone and a neurotransmitter.

4

Drugs that you too can understand if you really want to know. Just take a little bit more time.

4.1 Treatment for Epilepsy

Our brain is consisting of a complex network of neurons and their signals are transmitted via electric signal. However, when there is abnormal and excessive neuronal activity in the brain, symptoms such as seizures are likely to occur. It is a chronic neurological disorder that currently does not have a cure for it. Convulsion is a medical condition where muscles are uncontrolled shaking or contract. Some of the drugs treating epilepsy are anticonvulsants that try to suppress the excessive firing of neurons.

Here are the drugs to control epilepsy.

1. Sodium Valproate
This is an anticonvulsant that works by blocking the signal transmission located in the voltage-gated sodium channels and calcium channels and increases the level of GABA. GABA is gamma-aminobutyric acid that its primary function is to act as an inhibitory neurotransmitter in the central nervous system.

2. Carbamazepine
This is an anticonvulsant that works by stabilizing the inactivated state of sodium channels after it has sent a signal out by opening its channel.

3. Phenytoin
This drug treats chronic muscle spasm accompanies with pain. It works by stabilizing the inactivated state of sodium channels.

4. Ethosuximide
This is a T-type calcium channel blocker that helps to block signal from transmitting where T-type channel has awareness of time.

5. Phenobarbital

This is a barbiturate or depressant drug that has sedative and hypnotic properties. This activates GABA receptors and promotes GABA activity, and also blocks voltage-gated sodium channels.

6. Primidone

This drug usually is used for secondarily generalized seizures originating in the temporal lobes. It works by inhibiting action potentials generated by the voltage-gated sodium channels. It has a strong sedative effect so it is not the primary drug we use for treating epilepsy.

7. Clonazepam

This drug is like Primidone where it is also a secondary drug to use, and it sometimes uses with Primidone. It works by activating the GABA receptors which become more responsive to other neurons. As a result, synaptic transmission occurring in the central nervous system will be inhibited.

8. Gabapentin

This drug has a structure similar to GABA. However, many studies have shown that it may not act exactly as the natural GABA, but it does show to relieve pain. It may work by blocking the T-type calcium channels and by increasing the level of GABA.

4.2 Antibiotics

Infection is foreign substances invade the body, and most of time these foreign substances proliferate inside the body. Microorganisms like bacteria, fungi or infectious host-dependent agents such as virus can replicate themselves inside the body. Prion, however, is made of primarily protein and it does not self-replicate on its own and you probably never heard of it before, but surprisely you may have familiar with it if you have heard a disease called "mad cow disease".

Technically, antibiotics are drug kills microorganism, and antiviral is the drugs that kill virus, and antifungal are the drugs that kill fungus. Hopefully, this will clear up much confusion about why antibiotics do not destroy viruses.

The main actions of antibiotics are inhibiting the growth of bacteria when it begins to self-replicate.

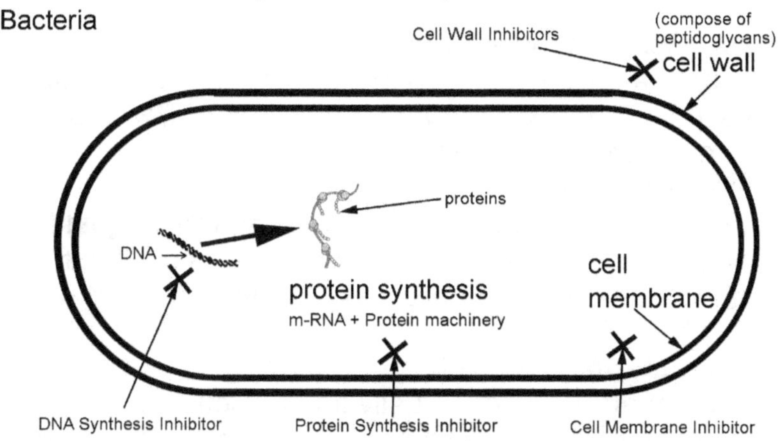

1. Beta-lactam Antibiotics – Cell Wall Inhibitors
Drugs like penicillin or cephems destroy the bacterial cell wall since its structure resemble to the component of cell wall called peptidoglycan, except it does not form cross-links with the other peptidoglycans to form the mesh-like layer. As a result, the cell wall is weaken and cause

rupture of cell wall when the bacteria cannot maintain a functional pressure again outside.

2. Cell Membrane Inhibitors

Polymyxin B is a good example in this class of drugs since it can bind to the bacterial cell membrane and disruptive the critical function of cell membrane for regulates what get inside and outside. As a result, cell membrane becomes more permeable and this leads to imbalance of ions and death.

3. Protein Synthesis Inhibitors

These drugs inhibit the growth of bacteria by disrupting the process of making new proteins. As you may know that proteins are synthesized in an assembly line fashion where the instruction was copied from the DNA via messenger-RNA and the message is transcribed and protein is synthesized. Tetracycline, as an example of these drugs, can inhibit the binding site of protein machinery, the ribosome permanently.

4. DNA Synthesis Inhibitors

Quinolone, a group of chemicals, is used to block bacterial DNA synthesis activity. Before a messenger-RNA can be produced from DNA, a specific section of DNA has to unwind. It's like before reading a page in a book, you need to open to that page, and unwinding DNA is just like opening a book to that page. Quinolone has ability of preventing the unwinding process in DNA.

5. Beta-lactamase Inhibitors

This type of drugs is not actually an antibiotic, but it does assist antibiotics to kill bacteria. Some bacteria become resistance against beta-lactam antibiotic because they are equipped with a new enzyme called beta-lactamase (penicillinase) that is capable of breaking the beta-lactam ring and these drugs become useless. However, a discovery was made to use beta-lactamase inhibitor such as clavulanic acid to assist with beta-lactam antibiotic to become effective in killing bacteria as it destroys the bacterial enzyme.

6. Mupirocin

This is an antibiotic that can treat methicillin-resistant staphylococcus aureus (MRSA)* which often infect on skin. However, it is used as topical. It acts on inhibiting RNA synthesis so no bacterial proteins can be produced. However, some studies have shown that staphylococcus may develop resistance against muprirocin.

*MRSA is also known as the "Super Bug"

7. Vancomycin

Methicillin-resistant staphylococcus aureus (MRSA) bacteria are almost always found to be resistant to multiple antibiotics. Treatment of MRSA by vancomycin has been reserved as a drug of "last resort" and it is used only after all other antibiotics had failed. It works by inhibiting cell wall synthesis by incorporate itself into the peptidoglycan cross-linked matrix. However, some bacteria began to show resistance against vancomycin as well.

8. Last Line of Defense against Bacterial Infection

Both linezolid and daptomycin are begun to be used as vancomycin becomes useless. Linezolid was introduced at 2009 as a newer synthetic antibiotic, and it acts as a protein synthesis inhibitor by disrupting the growth of bacterial protein. Daptomycin can destroy bacteria by disrupting many processes in the bacteria metabolism including its cell membrane function, DNA and RNA, and protein synthesis. It is a constant battle between man and bacteria as researchers searching for the next antibiotic.

4.3 Treatment for Parkinson's disease

Parkinson's disease (PD) is a result of the defect in dopamine production in the brain and the actual cause remains unknown. It's known that dopaminergic cells in the substantia nigra of the brain have reduced its productivity in secreting the dopamine. Dopamine acts as a neurotransmitter and a neurohormone that plays various roles in the brain and mainly the central nervous system.

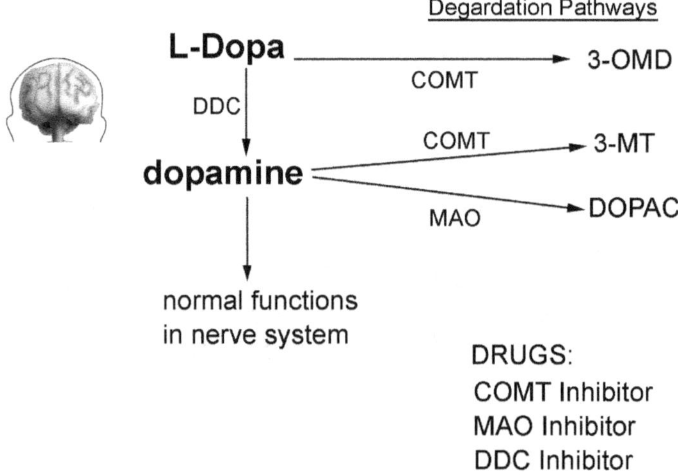

Here are drugs to treat Parkinson's disease and they mostly will try to increase the level of dopamine.

1. L-Dopa (Levodopa)

It's useless to supply more dopamine to the body since dopamine in the body cannot even enter into brain where it needed due to the presence of the blood-brain barrier. The precursor, L-Dopa, can enter it and convert into dopamine inside the brain and store in synaptic vesicles of synapse. In addition, L-Dopa is also administered with inhibitors such as the DDC and COMT inhibitors as we will discuss in next section.

2. Amantadine
This drug tends to promote the production of dopamine and the reabsorption of used dopamine. However, the exact mechanism is still under investigation. It's usually used in the early stages of disease.

3. Dopamine Agonists
These drugs bind to dopamine receptor and mimic the action of dopamine. Examples are pramipexole and ropinirole. In addition, a newer dopamine agonist called cabergoline has a long-acting effect as dopamine agonist and it can be administrated once a week.

4. Acetylcholine Inhibitors (Anticholinergic/Antimuscarinic Agents)
Both acetylcholine and dopamine should normally in a balance level but in patients with Parkinson's disease, the low level of dopamine make the effect of acetylcholine more appearance. As a result, patients are often developing tremors (shaking muscle) and stiffness which all relate to the imbalance of acetylcholine. An example of drugs is trihexyphenidyl hydrochloride, which classified as an antimuscarinic agent.

5. Adrenaline Precursors
The adrenal gland just located on the top of kidney secretes two important hormones called norepinephrine and epinephrine. These two hormones* also play important roles in the brain for increase the concentration of neurotransmitters in the body and brain. By taking drugs like droxidopa (L-DOPS), it can maintain the level of dopamine from degrading. In addition, L-DOPS is a man made adrenaline precursor that can enter into the blood-brain barrier and convert into norepinephrine and epinephrine inside the brain.

*Both norepinephrine and epinephrine have dual roles as a hormone and a neurotransmitter.

6. Monoamine Oxidase B Inhibitors (MAOI-Bs)
MAO found naturally in the body to degrade dopamine. Although there are two types, alpha and beta MAO, we use MAOI-beta inhibitor to inhibit the degradation of dopamine and increase the level of remaining dopamine. Examples are selegiline and rasagiline.

7. COMT (Catechol O-methyl Transferase) Inhibitors
They are a new type of medicines that stop the breakdown of dopamine. Since there are two normal pathways of degrading dopamine related to COMT pathway, one involves with DDC (dopa decarboxylase) and another involves with COMT (Catechol O-methyl Transferase). L-DOPA converts to dopamine by DDC or L-DOPA can be degraded by COMT into 3-OMD. Dopamine can be degraded by COMT.

These drugs inhibit COMT, so the level of dopamine and L-DOPA (if administrated) will increase. The reason we want to inhibit DDC as well is because that we want to preserve L-DOPA not to be degraded before it enters into the brain since dopamine itself cannot enter brain. Examples of COMT are entacapone and tolcapone. There are DDC inhibitors available as well, and they are carbidopa and benserazide.

4.4 Treatment for Rheumatoid Arthritis (RA)

Arthritis is still not a well known disease but it is believed that it is an autoimmune disease where the immune system is targeting at own tissues. Immune attack often leads to pain and inflammation in joints and these become life-long symptoms. Since there is no known cure for RA, two main treatments are available, where one aims for alleviate pain, and another aims for preventing irreversible damages.

Here are drugs to treat Rheumatoid Arthritis.

1. NSAIDs (See 2.7)
This is to alleviate the pain for RA by blocking the enzyme, COX that makes prostaglandins, which will help to reduce the pain. An example is diclofenac sodium.

2. Steroidal Anti-inflammatory Drugs
These drugs especially glucocorticoids can reduce inflammation by binding cortisol receptors which activates making more anti-inflammatory proteins. A good example will be prednisolone which is used to treat RA. In addition, steroidal drugs have additional effect on suppressing immune system by reducing the number of various immune cells.

3. Antirheumatic Drugs
These drugs like sodium aurothiomalate (which contains gold) or Gold Salt (ionic gold substance) can reduce inflammation and have longer effect.

4. Disease modifying anti-rheumatic drugs (DMARDs)
These drugs try to reduce the rate of damage done by RA in the areas of bone, cartilage, and joints. It is now recognized that the treatment of DMARDs is important in the early stages of disease since there was evidence suggested that joint damage happening in early stage as

well. An example of these drugs is methotrexate (as discussed in 1.3.3), which has shown to delay the structural damage in joint. Methotrexate acts as an inhibitor of DNA synthesis since it can inhibit the enzyme that make folic acid into the component of DNA, pyrimidine. In addition, methotrexate may also inhibit T cells from releasing interleukins and therefore preventing neutrophil to cause more damages to the tissue and inflammation. However, methotrexate is a toxic drug to be used.

4.5 Medication for Bronchitis

Treatment for bronchitis was to aim to open the airways from trachea into the lung in the past. However, until recently, it was recognized that bronchitis was most often caused by infection which resulted in inflammation and excessive secretion of mucus and led to narrowing the airways. Treatment for bronchitis is now aiming toward on reducing inflammation instead of just opening up the blockage.

Here are the treatments for bronchitis.

1. Beta-adrenergic Receptor Stimulant
This is one of the bronchodiating drugs which tend to increase the level of c-AMP and open airway in the lung. As level of c-AMP increases, it acts on dendritic cells in the immune system not to secrete that much mucus and less inflammation around the tissue in the lung. In short, it relaxes the smooth muscle and opens up the respiratory airways. Examples are beclometasone dipropionate and budesonide.

2. Theophylline
This is one of bronchodiating drugs widely used for treating asthma for many years. It acts by relaxing bronchial smooth muscle and also has some anti-inflammatory effect as it also promotes the level of c-AMP. It is naturally found in tea so that the name of this drug in many Asian countries contains the word tea in it. But the concentration of theophylline in tea does not reach to have any therapeutic doses. Many inhalers nowadays have replaced theophylline with anti-inflammatory steroids since theophylline had many side effects due to the fact it is very likely to interact with other drugs.

3. Steroidal Anti-inflammatory Drugs

These drugs are strong anti-inflammatory drugs that decreased inflammation and swelling by binding the cortisol receptor to increase more anti-inflammatory proteins. In addition, these drugs are now used in the inhaler since it only affects on the respiratory airways and didn't penetrate to body and induce side effects in the body. It can also be administrated by injection or orally.

4. Anticholinergic Agents
These drugs are usually used to treat chronic bronchitis, such as chronic obstructive lung disease (COLD). It blocks muscarinic cholinergic receptors and this will reduce the level of c-GMP, which indirectly inhibits constriction in airway smooth muscle. A good example of these drugs is ipratropium.

5. Anti-allergic Agents (Antihistamine)
These drugs are also used to treat bronchitis especially for the allergic bronchitis. Since allergic reaction begins when activating the histamine receptor H1 by the mast cells' releases of histamine in response to allergen (allergic substance). So by blocking the site of binding, it can reduce the level of allergic reactions. In addition, researches have shown that mast cells also play roles in regulating the airway smooth muscle functions. There are various groups of drug that targeting to reduce allergic reactions.

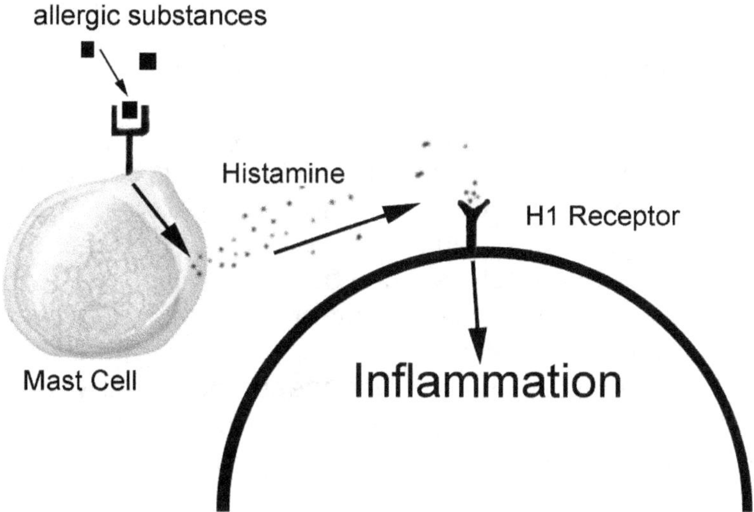

1. Anti-histamine (Mast Cells Stabilizers)
Drug like sodium cromoglicate inhibits the release of histamine from mast cells.

2. Anti-Leukotriene (Leukotriene Antagonist)
These drugs prevent inflammation in asthma and bronchitis by inhibiting the production of leukotrienes which induce inflammation effects. A good example is monteleukast.

3. Thromboxane Receptor Antagonist
These drugs treat chronic bronchitis by acting on thromboxane receptor. As discussed in the anti-thrombotic drugs in 3.8, thromboxane is necessary for blood aggregation. However, many researches have shown that there is a role of thromboxane A2 in setting a cough threshold where if the thromboxane receptor is deactivated by Thromboxane Receptor Antagonist, it can suppress the chronic coughing.* However, the exact mechanism is not clear at present time. An example of drugs is seratrodast.

** Involvement of thromboxane A2 in airway mucous cells in asthma-related cough*
http://jap.physiology.org/cgi/content/full/92/2/763

4. Anti-PAF (Platelet-activating factor)
These platelet-activating factors are produced in platelets, leukocytes (white blood cells), lung, and many other organs. These drugs can be used for treating bronchitis since besides activating the blood aggregation. Another function is to activate many types of leukocytes to initiate immune responses. By inhibiting these effects, airway inflammation will be reduced. An example of these drugs is epinastine.

5. Cytocine Inhibitors
This is a new type of anti-allergic agent as it acts on inhibiting the production of interleukin (IL) from the T-Cell helpers (Th-2 cells). An example of these drugs is suplatast tosilate*.

**FDA has not approved this type of drug, but it's developed and available in Japan since 1995.*

4.6 Sleep Aid and Anti-anxiety

Most of insomnia and excessive anxiety are usually accompanied with reasons and may not due to physical problems. However, in order to alleviate these suffering due to anxiety, many drugs are developed to help these conditions. These drugs are aiming at regulate nervous system's signals, but ultimately, one must find the reason that caused it initially in order to be independent from the drug's aid.

Here are the drugs for Anti-anxiety (anxiolytic).

1. Benzodiazepines (benzo)
This group of drugs all shares the same structure of a benzene ring and a diazepine. When people get excited or feel anxiety, various neurons are in excited state. The excited states are involved with various other elements, such as adrenaline, dopamine, and serotonin. By inhibiting these elements, one can alleviate symptoms of anxiety and insomnia. For example, the drug called chlordiazepoxide can act on GABA (inhibitory neurotransmitter as discussed in 4.1) in the benzodiazepine subreceptor. Once the level of GABA increases, it will inhibit dopamine-related signal pathway, adrenalin signals, and serotonin related signals.

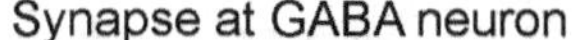

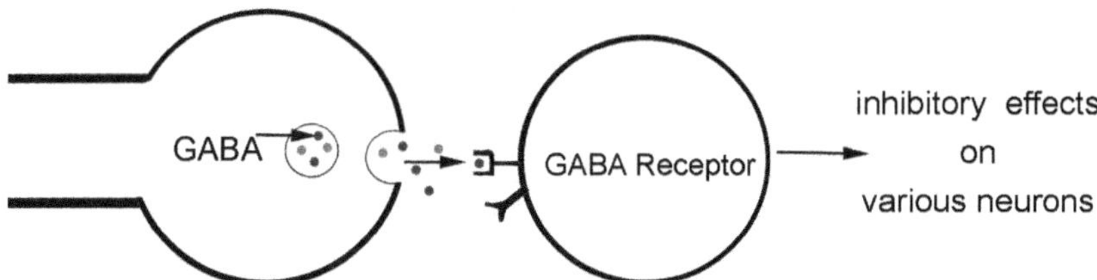

2. Tricyclin
As the name implies, it has a three-ring structure. Unlike benzodiazepines structurally, it has similar action similar to

benzodiazepines since it also acts on benzodiazepine subreceptor of the GABA. An example of these drugs is imipramine, which has been used for anxiety treatment for many years.

3. 5-HT1A Receptor Partial Agonists

A good example of these drugs is tandospirone*. Unlike previous drugs related to GABA's benzodiazepines' pathway, it acts on 5-HT1A Receptor of the serotonin (Section 1.4.3) and mediates the inhibitory neurotransmission. The disadvantage of using this drug is that it cannot last long in the body (shorter half-life). On the other hand, it has less side-effect.

*FDA has not approved this type of drug, but it's available in Japan since 1996 and also other countries.

4. Benzodiazepines as Sleep Aid

There are many Benzodiazepines used for treatment of insomnia and they are grouped into the degrees of how it lasts in the body. For example, fast acting but shorter effect one is trazolam, and short effect is brotizolam. Medium effect is flurazepam and lorazepam (Ativan)*, and longer-acting ones are nitrazepam and diazepam, which not recommended since they may persist into the next day.

*FYI: The mixture of lorazepam and propofol were found to be the reason caused the death of Michael Jackson in 2009.

4.7 Treatments for Depression

Patients suffer with depression have many different symptoms, such as difficulty concentrating, fatigue and no energy, and feeling of hopelessness. The causes of depression is complicated and related to both personalities and environments.

Patients diagnose with depression often are administrated with antidepressants. However, in fact antidepressants do not cure it, but will improve patients' conditions.

The biochemical theories explain the cause of depression is located in the synapse where either the number of neurotransmitters is less than normal or the number of receptors is more than necessary. Many drugs are developed based on these theories. These drugs are inhibiting the reuptakes of these neurotransmitters into the pre-synaptic cells. As results, the levels of these neurotransmitters are available to bind to the postsynaptic receptors.

1. Tricyclin (3 Rings, TCAs)
As discussed in 4.6.2, tricyclin is also used for increasing the level of monoamines, such as serotonin, norepinephrine, and dopamine). An example of these drugs is imipramine.

2. Tetracyclin (4 Rings, TeCAs)
These drugs have 4 rings structurally, and it has a similar effect as TCAs, and it also inhibits the reuptake of these monoamines, and the level of monoamines will be increased.

3. Serotonin-Specific Reuptake Inhibitors (SSRIs)
Both TCAs and TeCAs can affect the levels of serotonin, norepinephrine, and dopamine, but SSRIs can only affect serotoinin's reuptake. Therefore its effectiveness is not

comparable to TCAs or TeCAs, but it has less anticholinergic* side effects. Thus, it is still a widely used drug for treating depression. Examples** are fluvoxamine, paroxetine (Paxil), citalopram, fluoxetin (Prozac), dapoxetine, escitalopram, sertraline (Zoloft), and zimelidine.

* Anticholinergics are discussed in 4.5.4, and its side effects include loss of coordination, increase body temperature, and increase heart rate.

**Not all are FDA approved.

4. Serotonin-Norepinephrine Reuptake inhibitors (SNRIs)
In contrast to SSRIs, these drugs also work on inhibiting norepineprine's reuptake plus serotoinin's reuptake. It's a newer drug class than SSRIs and it has demonstrated to have higher antidepressant efficacy and fewer side effects compared to TCAs and TeCAs. Examples are desvenlafaxine, venlafaxine, tramadol, duloxetine, and bicifadine.

5. Monoamine Oxidase Inhibitors (MAOIs)
As discussed in 4.3.6, MAOI-Bs helps to increase the level of dopamine since it inhibits the MAO-beta particular affecting the dopamine's neurons. The MAOIs drugs are acting both MAO-alpha and MAO-beta to treat depression and anxiety since it prevents degradation of monoamine neurotransmitters, and as a result, it increases the availability. Examples of nonselective MAOIs are phenelzine (Nardil), harmine, hydralazine, nialamide, and safrazine. Since tyramine found in certain foods (such as cheese, avocados, soy products), patients taking MAOIs are advised not to eat it since it will dramatic increase blood pressure when tryramine interacts with MAOIs. Many antidepressants take a few weeks to achieve full therapeutic effects, and patients must be cautious not to interrupt these medications.

4.8 Antiarrhythmics

Treatments for irregular heart beat are also known as antiarrhythmics. Antiarrhythmics are extremely complicated and their mechanisms are difficult to simplify. In order to understand the drugs used for antiarrhythmics, we need to reference to Vaughan Williams (VW) classification which introduced in 1970. Sicilian Gambit's classification is based on VW and it's useful for clinical uses. There are five classes: I, II, III, IV, and V, and its mechanism of how drugs work relates to the location of action and clinical uses. These drugs commonly try to inhibit ion channels in the heart muscles in order to minimize the excessive heart beat.

Class I: Sodium (Na^{+}) Channel Blockers: disopyramide, pilsicainide hydrochloride, and lidocaine
Block Channels: Na

These drugs inhibit sodium ions from entering into heart muscle and prolong the time of action potential (Section 1.5) by extending the resting period that ready for the next nerve impulse. This class of drugs is also further divided into three subclasses: Ia, Ib, and Ic depending on its degree of actions on extending the resting period and how strong does it inhibit sodium channel.

Class II: Beta-blockers: propranolol, atenolol
Block Channels: Na, Ca

These drugs are beta-blockers that we have discussed in previous topics, such as lowering blood pressure, heart failure. Since it can block both sodium and calcium ion channels and it has the effects on blocking the catecholamines (Section 1.4.2), the heart rate can be controlled.

Class III: Extend Time for Repolarization: amiodarone, nifekalant, dofetilide
Block Channels: Na, Ca, K (potassium)

These drugs mainly block potassium channels and prolong the repolarization and increase the refractory period. All these contribute to prolong the time for the next round of nerve impulse to be fired.

Class IV: Slow Calcium (Ca^{2+}) Channel Blockers: diltiazem, verapamil
Block Channels: Ca, K

These drugs decrease the conduction via the AV node*, and shorten the next phase of cardiac action potential. Thus, these drugs can also inhibit the concentration of calcium ions from rising in the heart muscle cells and reduce the chance of being excessive excitement for the heart muscle cells. Thus, these drugs are able to control both the heart rate and heart's contractility.

*The heart beat begins with Sinoatrial node (SA node) located at the top of heart and when the pulse travel to center of heart, the atrioventricular node (AV node) send another impulse to the entire heart. This second impulse made by AV node has a normal delay of 0.12 second since it allows the atria to have total ejected their blood into the ventricles before the ventricles contract. If it's too fast, arrhythmias will be resulted.

Class V: Other Agents: Unknown mechanism: digoxin, adenosine
Block Channels: N/A

This class was added to VW's original classification for those drugs that does not fit into classes I to IV. For example, adenosine reduces the level of cAMP and thus temporary cause a block in the AV node. Digoxin, on the other hand, increases the vagal activity* and then reduces the conductivity on the AV node since it can act on the central nervous system directly.

*Vagal activity refers to the activity on the vagus nerve which is a nerve system that is located around the ear and jaw and extend all the way to the heart. Vagus nerve mediates the parasympathetic part of the heart and affects the heart by slowing down.

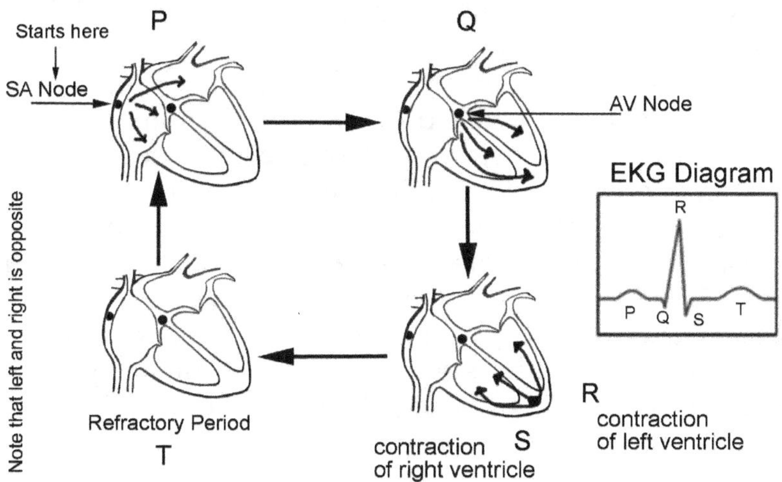

Visual animation illustration:
http://www.nhlbi.nih.gov/health/dci/Diseases/hhw/hhw_electrical.html

4.9 Analgesic

These drugs are also known as painkiller. The experience of pain can be divided into two groups. One is the cause of the pain at the local site. Another is the signal of pain received in the brain. Analgesic focuses on blocking the signal passes to the brain. Here are the analgesic drugs.

1. Non-Steroidal Anti-Inflammatory Drugs (NSAIDs) (See Section 2.7)

One of most popular over the counter drugs is acetaminophen and it acts on COX enzyme that responsible for synthesis of prostaglandins. Reduction in the level of prostaglandins will reduce the symptoms of pain, fever, and inflammation. However, the degree of reducing these symptoms varies among drugs in this drug class. Since many NSAIDs are not selective on COX-2, it inhibits COX-1 as well. As results, they inhibit normal bodily functions in platelets, blood vessels, and kidney. For example, one of adverse side effects from acetaminophen is liver damage.

2. Opiates

There are many opioid receptors in the body, which located in central nerve system and along the intestinal nerves. There are four major types of opioid receptors: delta, kappa, mu, and OP4, and where mu receptors have better effect on strong pain, respiratory controls, and euphoria. Both morphine and codeine can be extracted from the opium (poppy) plant. Morphine acts directly on the central nervous system to relieve pain by binding* to mu-receptor but it does not last long since it has a short half-life. Codeine can be produced from morphine, and it only has 2 to 25 percent the strength of morphine since everyone has different sensitivity and metabolism rate toward it. In low dose, codeine is used in suppressing cough. Unfortunately, all opiates have shown to cause physical dependence with long-term intake.

*Morphine will be breakdown into a form that can bind to the mu-receptor.

Meditation

Many researches now show promising results for practicing meditation for treating patients with chronic pain. Some patients are able to relax their minds and learn not to depend on painkiller. One of reasons that these opiates can cause dependency is because the body stops producing endorphins, a natural pain reliever in the body, when opiates enter into body system.

4.10 Medication for Cancer

Research into the treatment of cancer can be dated back at least 80 years ago, but we still do not have effective medication for treating and curing cancer because cancerous cells were developed from the normal cells. Drugs used to treat cancer can be grouped into two groups. One is aiming at damaging and killing the cancer cells, and another is to specifically target the substances (which are unique only to cancerous cells) inside the cancer cells.

Attack Targets on Cancer Cells

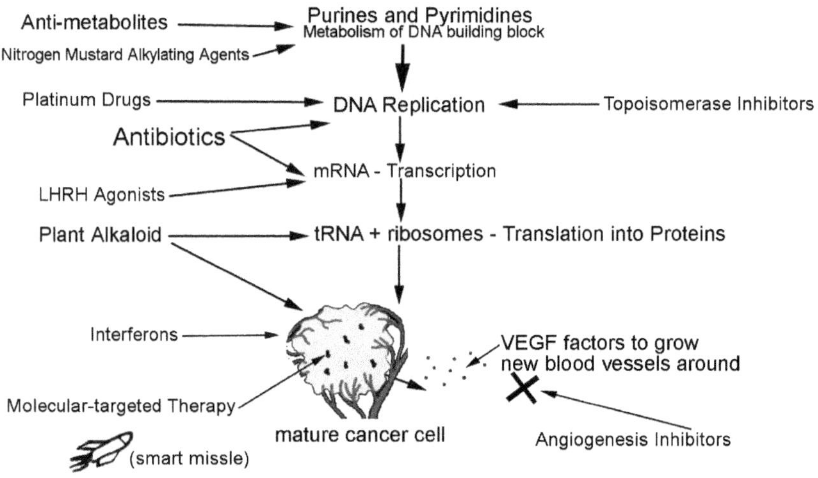

Drugs for Killing Cancer Cells

1. Nitrogen Mustard Alkylating Agents*
These drugs are alkylating agent which can attach an alkyl group to DNA specifically the guanine base of DNA. However, because of its non-selective action, they are toxic to normal cells as well. Replication will be impossible since DNA is basically stuck since its strands are unable to uncoil properly. Examples are melphalan, cyclophosphamide, and nimustine hydrochloride.

*These agents were the infamous chemical weapons used in World War I as the “mustard gas”.

2. Anti-metabolites

These drugs aim at affecting the DNA and RNA synthesis since these agents mainly prevent the building blocks of DNA or RNA from incorporating. For examples, as discussed in 1.3.3 and 4.4.4, methotrexate is a drug that prevents the dihydrofolic acid reductase enzyme from converting diydrofolate into tetrahydrofolate and eventually affecting the conversion of dUMP* into dTMP*, nucleic acids necessary to synthesize pyrimidine**, a component of DNA. Methotrexate has a similar structure as folic acid and it inhibits the enzyme by binding to it as antagonist. Other examples are fluorouracil and mercaptopurine. Fluorouracil inhibits thymidylate synthase and mercaptopurine competes with the normal purine to form AMP and GMP.

*dUMP is deoxyuridine monophosphate and dTMP is deoxythymidine monophosphate
**There are two components that made up the DNA: Purines (Adenine, Guanine) and Pyrimidines (Cytosine, Thymine)

3. Antibiotics that used as chemotherapeutic

Drugs like mitomycin C is able to form crosslink with DNA and therefore inhibits DNA synthesis. Doxorubicin can fit between pairs of DNA and inhibits DNA replication. This is used in Hodgkin’s lymphoma.

4. Plant Alkaloid

Vincristine is from vinca plant, and it acts as a mitotic inhibitor. As a result, it prevents cells from undergoing mitosis or cell division where it disrupts the microtubule formation that is necessary for cell pulling away from each other to form two cells. In contrast, paclitaxel stabilizes microtubules and prevents it from degrading in order to enter the next phase of cell division.

5. Platinum-containing Drugs
Cisplatin uses its platinum to bind DNA by forming a crosslink and this will trigger apoptosis at the end. Other examples are carboplatin and nedaplatin

6. Hydrolysis Enzymes
Drug like L-asparaginase can be used to treat acute lymphoblastic leukemia since leukemic cells are just like other normal cells need nutrients like amino acid asparagines but unlike normal cells, they cannot make their own asparagines. Therefore, by destroying the circulating asparagines with asparainase, leukemic cells will die from starving as asparagines convert asparagines to aspartic acid.

7. Endocrine Therapy with Luteinizing Hormone-Releasing Hormone (LHRH) Agonists
Some cancer cells are hormone dependent which are called hormone-responsive cancers. For an example, breast cancer cells* require estrogen to grow. By combining both anti-estrogen (tamoxifen) and anti-steroidal agent (exemestane), it can lower the source of estrogens. Tamoxifen works by binding to estrogen receptor as antagonist and prevents estrogen from binding the receptors on the breast tissue. Exemestane works by permanently bind to enzyme that converts androgens into estrogens. Another example will be leuprorelin acetate. It acts at pituitary GnRH receptors, which results in down regulates the secretion of luteinizing hormone (LH) and follicle-stimulating hormone (FSH) in women for treating breast and ovarian cancer and suppress testosterone production in men for treating advanced prostate cancer.

*Cancer cells may share the same name, like breast cancer, but they do not necessary behave the same. So breast cancer can be further divided into hormone-responsive and hormone-nonresponsive.

8. Topoisomerase Inhibitors

Since topoisomerase is responsible for cutting and reanneling* DNA and unwinding DNA strands in order for DNA to replicate and transcribe. Topoisomerase is essential for cell growth and protein synthesis. These drugs prevent DNA from unwinding and thus block DNA replication. Irinotecan is a topoisomerase 1 inhibitor, which inhibits the cut of one strand of a DNA double helix. Etoposide is a topoisomerase 2 inhibitor, which inhibits the cut of both strands of a DNA double helix

*Reanneal is to form duplex DNA or the process of combining two single strands of DNA into double-stranded DNA.

9. Angiogenesis Inhibitors

Cancer that forms solid mass need nutrients to grow, so cancer cells are able to grow new blood vessels around them (angiogenesis) and draw nutrients to themselves. Antiangiogenic drugs prevent the Vascular Endothelial Growth Factor (VEGF) from binding the receptors on endothelial cells since these cells are responsible for growing new walls of blood vessels. This treatment takes advantage of the fact that adult body does not make new vessels unless there is active tissue repair. Examples of these drugs are bevacizumab and carboxyamidotriazole.

10. Interferons (IFN)

These substances are naturally occurring proteins produce in the body. It is part of body's immune system against viral infection. There are many types of interferon, where IFN–alpha is produced by leukocytes, IFN-beta is produced by fibroblasts, and IFN-gamma produced by lymphocytes. They work like a signal system where the immune system can identify the target and destroy it. Drug like Multiferon can be used for treating cutaneous melanoma. Other drugs like Imidazoquinoline are able to induce the production of IFN-alpha.

Molecular-targeted Therapy for Cancer

In this type of medication, it attempts to block the growth of cancer by targeting specific molecules inside the cancer. In order for cancerous cells to grow and spread inside the body, they rely on their own signaling pathways. This therapy attempts to first identify the substance that mediates the signaling, and then target to interfere it. As a result, this will block the signals that tell cancer cells to grow and it may lead to apoptosis as discussed in 3.5.3. Other method of targeted therapy may directly cause the cancer cell to die by delivering toxic substances to them as a silver bullet.

1. Gefitinib
This drug is an EGFR* inhibitor that targets for interfering the EGFR in malignant cells.

* EGFR is epidermal growth factor receptors that are located on the surface of cell and play roles in cell proliferation and DNA synthesis.

2. Trastuzumab
This drug is a monoclonal antibody that gathers around the HER2/neu receptor that embedded in cell membrane of the cancer cells, and this is to block the communication between cancer cells.

3. Imatinib Mesilate (Novartis or Gleevec in US)
This drug is a tyrosine kinase inhibitor and also used for treating chronic myelogenous leukemia (CML) since it inhibits bcr-abl proteins, which were developed from a mutation in the chromosome. In detail, bcr-abl protein is an abnormal tyrosine kinase which is always in "ON" mode so it keeps activating a number of cell cycle-controlling proteins and enzymes. By inhibiting this abnormal protein, cell division will be in controlled.

Additional Sources Treatments of Cancer

www.cancer.gov
www.acor.org
http://cancer.about.com
www.oncologychannel.com
www.soifind.com/searchweb.aspx?q=cancer+treatments
www.cancer.org

Conclusion

Our mind is the most powerful medicine of all. Have you ever heard the placebo effect? Placebo effect is a phenomenon that patients actually feel better when they receive “sugar pill” that does not have therapeutic effect, but patients do not know about it. And do you know fear can cause health problems or even lead to death? There was a story during World War II that a prisoner was tied and blindfolded. When someone scratched his wrist and told him that he would bleed to death and then let him hear the sound of water drips from the faucet. The man soon died from his own fear. These all prove that the mind is extremely powerful.

Your thoughts may lead to different outcomes. After reading this book, I hope that you have new understandings about the intricate biochemistry happening inside your body and you will appreciate life much more. Since those biochemistry reactions are not merely chemical reactions, ultimately, it is you and your body fighting illness together! You are the last line of defense.

So take care of your body seriously. Do you know learning a new exercise can boost your energy level? To keep a healthy body, it’s not necessary to do strenuous exercises or even join a gym. Regular exercise with sensible nutrition is the key for a healthier body. Why not try to learn meditation? It’s a workout for the mind! See how exercise both the mind and body can benefit you.

Appendix I: Prescription abbreviations used by medical professionals

You can learn to understand those commonly used abbreviations based on Latin words on your prescription that doctor prescribed to you after a doctor's visit.

Abbreviation / Meaning / Latin

Aa /of each/ ana
Ad/ up to / ad
a.c. /Before meals/ Ante cibum
a.d./ right ear/ aurio dextra
ad.lib. /use as much as one wants /Ad libitum
admov/ apply / admove
agit/ stir or shake / agita
alt. h. / every other hour / alternis horis
a.m. / morning, before noon / alternis meridiem
aq. /Water /Aqua
b.i.d. /Twice a day /Bis in die
b.i.n. /Twice a night/ Bis in noctus
c / with bar on top /With /Cum
c / food / cibos
cap. /Capsule /Capula
cc / with food / cum cibos
cr., crm/ cream
cf / with food /
d /Day /Dies
daw /Dispense as written(no generic)
div. /Divide /Divide
eq.pts. /Equal parts /Equalis parties
gtt or gt /Drop /Gutta
h. /Hour /Hora
h.s. (hs) /Bedtime /Hora somni
ID / intradermal
I.M. /Into the muscle
I.V. /Into the vein

IVP / intravenous push
mg /Milligram
ml /Milliliter
no. /Number /Numero
noxt /At night
o. /Pint /Octarius
O.D. /Right eye /Oculo dextro
O.S. /Left eye /Oculo sinistro
O.U. /In each eye /Oculo utro
p.c. /After meals /Post cibum
p.m./ evening or afternoon / post meridiem
p.o. /By mouth /Per os
p.r.n. /As needed /Pre re nata
pulv / powder / pulvis
pil /Pill /Pilula
q 1 d /Every day /Quaque 1 die
q 1 w /Once a week
q 3 h /Every 3 hours /Quaque 3 hora
q.i.d. /4 times a day /Quarter in die
q.o.d. /Every other day
q.s. /Sufficient quantity /Quantum sufficiat
qAM/ Every morning
qd /Daily /Quaque die
qh /Every hour /Quaque hora
R / rectal
Rep / repeat / repetatur
s /Without Sine
s.i.d. /Once a day /Semel in die
s.l. /Under the tongue
Sig., S. /Write on the label /Signa
stat /Immediately /Statim
tab /Tablet /Tabella
tbsp /Tablespoon
tid /3 times a day /Ter in die
top / topical
tr, tinc / tincture
tsp /Teaspoon
ut dict /As directed by doctor
ung / ointment / unguentum

U.S.P / United States Pharmacopoeia
vag / vaginally
w / with
w/o / without
X / times
Y.O. / years old

INDEX

About the Author

Arthur Wang received a degree in biochemistry from UCLA. He also had extensive studies in microbiology, immunology, western medicine and traditional Chinese medicine. He is also an enthusiastic writer on various topics on the internet. Besides working, he has been actively involved in volunteer work for many years. Arthur Wang lives and works in Los Angeles, California.

http://what-doctors-are-prescribing.blogspot.com

www.ingramcontent.com/pod-product-compliance
Lightning Source LLC
LaVergne TN
LVHW020647100826
845148LV00012B/2363
* 9 7 8 0 9 8 2 6 3 4 7 0 7 *